The International Library of Psychology

THE DEVELOPMENT OF THE SEXUAL IMPULSES

Founded by C. K. Ogden

The International Library of Psychology

PHYSIOLOGICAL PSYCHOLOGY
In 10 Volumes

THE DEVELOPMENT OF THE
SEXUAL IMPULSES

R E MONEY-KYRLE

First published in 1932 by
Routledge

Reprinted in 1999 by
Routledge
2 Park Square, Milton Park, Abingdon, Oxon, OX14 4RN

Transferred to Digital Printing 2007

British Library Cataloguing in Publication Data
A CIP catalogue record for this book
is available from the British Library

The Development of the Sexual Impulses
ISBN 0415-21078-X
Physiological Psychology: 10 Volumes
ISBN 0415-21131-X
The International Library of Psychology: 204 Volumes
ISBN 0415-19132-7

CONTENTS

CONTENTS ix

THE DEVELOPMENT OF THE SEXUAL IMPULSES

PREFACE

My original motive for writing this book was an intellectual discomfort, a desire to clear my mind and to bring some order and consistency into my ideas about psycho-analysis and the relations of this science to philosophy,physiology, biology, anthropology, sociology and ethics. I hope it may possibly satisfy a similar desire in some of those who read it. If it contains anything original this is to be found more in its form than in its content. The subjects with which it deals are usually presented in isolation, so that their intimate relations with each other are not easily perceived. The aim of this work is to present them in one system and thereby to give a general and consistent impression of the wood which an exclusive attention to the individual trees has often made so obscure.

No one can speak authoritatively on more than one science. But unfortunately no science is independent of others—least of all psychology. In an age of over-specialization the defects in a work which has its roots in so many sciences may be forgiven, when it is remembered that its author is prevented by the variety of his subjects from being a specialist in any of them.

The first chapter is devoted to what may be called the philosophy of psychology. If it is dull and unintelligible, the author is to blame. But those who think that the subject is itself irrelevant should remember that most physicists of the nineteenth century thought philosophy irrelevant. In reality they were encumbered by the philosophy of common sense, and the extraordinary advance which their science has since made was due to the revolt against this attitude led by men like Gauss, Helmholtz and Mach, who paved the way for Einstein. And Einstein himself is said to have been reading Hume at the time he made that first renunciation of the prejudices of common sense which culminated in the theory of relativity.

Like the physics of a bygone age the psychology of the present day is still encumbered with a mixture of dualistic materialism and animistic spiritualism which must be eliminated before there can be any comparable advance. One type of psychology is indeed free from this reproach, but it has shirked, not solved its difficulties by limiting its scope to the field of observable behaviour. I have tried to present a conception of psychology which reconciles Behaviourism with Introspection and combines the merits of both.

When the primitive ideas in any science have been

tidied up, the next stage is to systematize the body of doctrine it contains. A few propositions are selected to form the apex of an inverted pyramid and the rest are shown to be logically deducible from these. It is obvious that psychology is not ripe for the completion of this process, but at least a suggestion can be made of the outlines that the finished structure is likely to assume. If we cannot prove that the more complex processes we believe we find follow logically from the simpler ones of which we are sure, we can at least show that they are not incompatible, and that they are the sort of results which we ought to expect.

This kind of argument seems to be not only possible but also desirable in psychology and especially in the psychology of the psycho-analytic school. Belief may be founded either on personal experience or on a train of deduction. At the present moment the evidence which psycho-analysts can bring to support their theories is almost always an appeal to personal experience. Personal experience may be the only certain proof, but the kind to which psycho-analysts refer is very difficult to obtain. And, since the assertions they make are also unpalatable, it is not surprising that they are seldom believed. Psycho-analysts cannot analyse the whole world, or even a majority of its population, so that if they desire that their science should be accepted and have a chance of exercising the influence it should have, it will be necessary for them to find some argument other than the appeal to personal experience.

If it is not yet possible to deduce psycho-analytic

prepositions from simpler propositions of psychology which everyone would accept, I believe it could nevertheless be shown that they are at least plausible consequences of what is already known or suspected in physiology, biology, and anthropology. The greater part of this book is an attempt to indicate the lines on which this might be done.

Thus in Chapter II I have tried to formulate the simplest psychological mechanisms from which the more complex processes disclosed by psycho-analysis can be composed. In Chapter III I have tried to suggest how evolution may have elaborated some of these higher mechanisms, and in Chapter IV how culture may have elaborated others. In Chapter V I have tried to outline a psycho-analytic view of the development of the individual. Even if there is little that is original in my account of the evolution of instincts, the growth of culture, and the development of the individual, I hope that by juxtaposing outlines of these three forms of development they may be made to illuminate each other.

The last chapter is concerned with the effect and value of psychology. Socrates gave the world the command ' Know thyself ' ; and, since he assumed further that all moral error was ultimately due to intellectual error, he supposed that everything would be perfect in a world whose citizens had a complete knowledge of psychology. Admittedly Plato in the *Republic* qualified this view and allowed only the Guardians to be wholly wise. But we shall be more uncompromising than Plato and try to foresee some of the aspects of a completely enlightened world. We shall probably find that complete self-knowledge is impossible for the human species, and that indeed some irrationality is necessary for its continued existence.

It is necessary to say a word about the system of numbering the paragraphs in this Book. Roman numerals stand for chapters and Arabic numerals for sections and sub-sections. The first digit stands for a section, the second for a sub-section, and so on. Thus ' iii. 214 ' refers to chapter iii, section 2, sub-section 1, sub-sub-section 4. References are given to sections and not to pages.

Lastly I wish to record my gratitude to Dr. Ernest Jones, Prof. Flügel, Dr. C. P. Blacker and my wife for reading the whole or portions of the manuscript and for making many valuable criticisms and suggestions.

CHAPTER I

The Nature of Psychology

1. Interactionism and Behaviourism.

The psychology of the present day is necessarily a hybrid science whose parents are introspection and the study of behaviour. For we are not yet able either fully to systematize our mental lives without some reference to the physical processes of stimulus and reaction, or adequately to explain behaviour in terms of neural processes without some reference to mental states. The usual procedure is to give mental causes for behaviour and physical causes for thought, or in other words, to treat consciousness as an intermediary cause between stimuli and reactions.

Thus ordinary psychology seems to imply a dualistic interactionist philosophy. This philosophy regards the consciousness and the body as belonging to two separate kinds of reality, which interact upon each other. Thus the consistent interactionist must suppose that, although in simple reflexes the reaction is physically determined by the stimulus and by the engrams of former stimuli, the mechanical chain of processes of more complex reflexes is sometimes interrupted by a mental link

6

of a heterogeneous substance which is at least partially determined by the receptor stimulus and at least partially determines the muscular response. Most psychologists are untroubled by the philosophical assumptions of their science and are content to go their way without either questioning them or following up their further implications. Dr. Watson, however, has been so disturbed by these assumptions that he appears to have denied consciousness altogether in order to limit psychology to Behaviourism. And Prof. McDougall has applied a dualistic interactionist conception to maintain the partial independence of the soul. For, once the mind is believed to break the physical causal chain from stimulus to behaviour, it is easy to go on to state that the mind is only partially determined by receptor stimulus and that it is open to other influences, such as the voice of God, or that it is partly 'free'.

Now I believe that the procedure of ordinary psychology is legitimate, but that the philosophical conception which seems to justify it is misleading. It has led both to the behaviouristic repudiation of the method of ordinary psychology and to the interactionist denial of the physical determinateness of behaviour. Such results seem deplorable ; for I believe that these two sciences should be each other's closest allies. I propose here to submit a concept of the nature of psychology which reconciles the claims of both. But I shall start with the apparently irrelevant questions : How is physics constructed ? And how is it applied ?

B

8 DEVELOPMENT OF SEXUAL IMPULSES

2. The construction of physics.[1]

In the terminology of Hume, consciousness may be divided into impressions and ideas, or, what is the same thing, into sensations and images.[2] These differ from one another in distinctness and in other characteristics enumerated by him. The most important difference is that ideas are more directly dependent on wishes than are impressions. Ideas are reproductions of impressions, and impressions are patterns of colours, sounds, tactual sensa and the like.

The visual field of the child may be supposed to consist at first almost wholly of sensations. Among these, certain sensa-complexes are relatively stable and form the core of what are later called material objects. And among these again are some which are more or less permanent constituents of the foreground. These are later distinguished from other material objects as parts of the self.[3]

Visual contact between part of the self (that is a constituent of the permanent foreground of the field of view) and any of those relatively stable complexes we call sense objects is invariably accompanied by a sensation of hardness. Further, contact between two objects of the environment is visually similar to contact between the hand and one of these ; it evokes therefore

[1] This section is mainly taken, by the kind permission of the Editor, from my paper " Belief and Representation " published in *Symposion*, 1927.

[2] Each of these concepts may be regarded as the limit of a process of abstraction.

[3] Mach, *Die Analyse der Empfindungen*, i.

the image which is the copy of the tactual sensa that would have accompanied this. Finally any visual object, even when not in contact with anything, excites the idea of hardness. That is, we feel empathetically what happens to other objects as though it had happened to ourselves. And, even when nothing is happening to them, we see them only together with the image of that feeling of solidity which varies, but never completely disappears, with the violence of the events in which our own body is seen to play a part. Thus in the perceptual field visual objects are fringed with tactual memories.

21. *The world of common sense.*

Memories or reproductions of former perceptual fields may be pieced together in the order in which they originally occurred. Such an ideal construction, resembling an amplified perceptual field, forms what we call the external world of common sense. Because it is composed of ideas rather than sensations, any part of it can come into being when and as we choose, with or without that foreground which we call ourselves. In this sense, unlike the perceptual field, it exists independently of us, independent alike of our movement and our presence. Any particular field of view corresponds to some part of this external world ; it is the original of which this is a copy ; and as sensations vary, lighting up now this, now that part of the ideal extension of our environment, we say that we are moving in the external world from place to place.

22. The world of physics.

Just as the external world of common sense is the ideal *extension* of our perceptual field, so is the world of physics the ideal *refinement* of the world of common sense.

That half-circle of continuous green we call a distant tree is seen on a close inspection to be composed of a multitude of leaves ; and we ever after speak of this sensa-complex as being always there waiting to be seen, as being the real tree of which the half-circle of continuous green is but the appearance. It is permanently there in the sense that its memory image is a constituent of our world of common sense. Thus the difference between appearance and reality is the difference between a sensa-complex as seen from afar and the memory of what this complex changed into when we approached it closely.

The analogy of the tree suggests that a still closer inspection of the leaves would change them also into an atomic structure. Microscopic inspection verifies this anticipation, and chemistry enables us to guess at what might be seen or felt beyond the limits of the microscope. And in this way the atomic world of nineteenth century physics was constructed. It was believed to be real in the sense that every part of it was believed to be a theoretical possibility of experience.

But this mechanistic physical world was found to be less satisfactory than was at first supposed. The grosser physical changes of liquids that boiled or froze could be accounted for along these lines ; that is, they could be correlated with a simple mechanistic picture. But some of the mutual interdependences of objects at a distance from each other eluded the attempt to correlate them with mechanistic pictures. Finally it was found more convenient to substitute for this atomic world a purely mathematical construction. The four dimensions of the world of common sense can be correlated with four series of real numbers, a point with an ordered set of four numbers, one chosen from each of the four series ; the characteristics of the point with another set called potentials ; and the laws of nature by relations between the potentials of neighbouring points. Thus the world of physics of the present day is a purely mathematical construction from which every other quality has been abstracted. For it is a peculiarity of the scientific world that the number of its distinct qualities decreases as it is refined. The table of the perceptual field and of the world of common sense is hard and coloured ; the physical table is at first composed of particles that are hard and energetic, but which possess no colour, and later of a colony of places where the measurement of the angles of triangles give strange results.

But though the physical world is ultimately a conceptual world it is not arbitrary. It is formed by definite rules of abstraction, interpolation, and extrapolation, operating upon the perceptual field. It is even objective in a certain sense. For if the same operations of abstraction, interpolation, and extrapolation are performed on different perceptual fields, the same physical world results. The physical world is real in the sense that it is objective, that is, common to all observers.

3. *The relation of the physical world to consciousness.*

The physical world is thus ultimately a conceptual world, a mathematical construction. It is an idea of man and is therefore not a reality separate from the reality of consciousness but a part of the consciousness of the scientist who thinks it. And even if it stands for a reality beyond, this can only be another perceptual world theoretically possible to beings with more sensitive sense organs— not something which exists independently of being seen. Thus, when we speak of real objects, as opposed to sensations of them, we mean the conceptual object which the operation of physical abstraction applied to the sense object would yield. Since the physical world is not a reality separate from consciousness, but an abstraction from consciousness, relations between it and consciousness are not relations between two separate realities but relations between concepts and feelings. For this reason the dualistic-interactionist basis of ordinary psychology is misleading, even if, for reasons which will presently appear, its consequences are often true.

4. *The applications of physics.*

The object of science is to give knowledge, that is, true expectations of experience. By itself that construction which is the physical world gives no knowledge

and is entirely useless ; but there are certain procedures
by which true expectations can be calculated from it.
These are mainly of three kinds, and form three branches
of applied physics which we will consider in turn.

41. *Inverted physics.*

The first makes use of the correlation between
physical objects and external sensations, and may be
called inverted physics, for it inverts the process by
which the physical world was originally constructed.
The physical world is an abstraction from the world
of common sense and is therefore correlated with it.
Thus, to find out what any part of the common sense
world would look like, it is only necessary to reverse
that process by which the physical world was constructed.   Now the common sense world is formed by
piecing together our memories, and is therefore small
in space and time, and full of gaps.   But the physical
world is uniform, so that we can extrapolate it beyond
the boundaries of the common sense world and inter-
polate its gaps.   Thus, if we want to know what the
common sense world would look like beyond our
experience we can construct it from the physical world,
which is larger and more complete, by reversing the
same process of abstraction which we applied to that
part of the common sense world which came within
our experience.   In other words we know that physics
would reduce a certain sensa-complex in the common
sense world first to a collection of atoms and finally
to a piece of world geometry, so that, if another part
of the physical world is similarly constructed, we know

that the corresponding perceptual field would contain a similar sensa-complex.

Inverted physics is therefore the procedure by which we can extend the sense world beyond our fields of view. But it can only tell us what external sensations to expect, and not the emotions and ideas that will be associatively evoked by these. Thus, if inverted physics were the only kind of applied physics, the world of physics would be of no use in helping us to anticipate any experience except external sensations. But even these external sensations would not be definitely foretold. Inverted physics only tells us what sensa-complexes we should have if certain conditions (which it does not itself specify) were fulfilled. There must be no impervious matter between the place in the physical world which corresponds to these sensa-complexes in the common sense world, and our sense organs, and no break in the neural path from these sense organs to the brain. Thus, inverted physics specifies correlations between the world of physics and certain *possibilities* of sensation, that is, it specifies correlations which do not hold good unconditionally, but only under conditions which it is beyond its scope to specify.

42. *Physiological psychology.*

The second type of applied physics makes use of a correlation between sensory stimuli and sensations. It is the science of physiological psychology. We know that retinal impressions, if the brain and nerves are intact, usually give rise to visual impressions. And similar receptor-sensory relations hold for all the external sense organs of the body. Thus, physiological psychology can, theoretically at least, give us all the true expectations that we can obtain from inverted physics. But it gives us more than this. For there are internal sense organs as well as external. We know, for instance, that certain visceral stimuli give rise to sensations of hunger, and it has been argued that all emotions are visceral sensations. Thus, physiological psychology can theoretically give true expectations about both external and internal sensations, whereas inverted physics only gives information about external sensations. But like inverted physics, physiological psychology does not specify unconditional correlations. It states what sensations would be correlated with what stimuli if the neural path from the sense organs to the brain is unbroken by physical injury or central inhibition. Its degree of indeterminateness is, however, less than that of inverted physics ; for, whereas inverted physics assumes unspecified conditions both between external objects and sense organs, and between sense organs and brain, physiological psychology only assumes the second of these two.

43. *Psycho-physics.*

The third type of applied physics, which can be called psycho-physics, is not yet far advanced, but if it were ever completed it would render the other two theoretically unnecessary. It investigates a direct correlation between cerebral processes[1] and consciousness. This

---

[1] Or perhaps it would be safer to say ' nervous processes in the " sensorium " ' instead of ' cerebral processes.'

correlation is probably, unlike those investigated by inverted physics and physiological psychology, not only valid for the whole of consciousness, instead of for the sensory part alone, but also unconditioned by unspecified assumptions concerning the environment of the organism or the state of its nervous system. Thus, if psycho-physics is ever wholly successful in its task a complete knowledge of the state of the brain would enable the scientist of the future to calculate the complete state of the corresponding consciousness. Thus, if the two sciences of physics and psycho-physics could be completed, the one to determine the precise condition of a given brain and the other to determine the psychological correlates of this condition, any sensation, feeling, or idea which will occur or has occurred could be foretold or reconstructed. Then science would be omniscient. But we cannot hope, and we need not fear, that it will more than approximate to this ideal

5. *Psychology.*

We are now in a better position to form a concept of the nature of psychology which will justify its procedure without admitting the implications of a dualistic interactionism. Psychology is not only Behaviourism, for this is a branch of physics that takes no account of consciousness, nor is it only Introspection, for it makes repeated reference to the physical 'causes' and 'effects' of mental processes, nor again is it purely psycho-physics, for it is not confined to the determination of the psychical correlates of cerebral events. I think that ultimately it will be regarded as a combination of Behaviourism and Psycho-physics, which is charged with the dual problem of working out the causes and effects of cerebral processes in stimuli and reactions, and of correlating these processes with conscious states. It will investigate at once the causal chain ' *stimulus—cerebral process—reaction* ' and the correlation ' *cerebral process—consciousness.*' Thus the connections and relations which it will study may be represented diagramatically as follows :

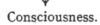

Stimulus→Cerebral Process→Reaction
↓
Consciousness.

This formulation of the problems of psychology seems to me to bring out clearly that both Interactionism and Behaviourism are right in what they affirm and wrong in what they deny. In virtue of the one-one correlation which we assume to exist between cerebral processes and consciousness, the two expressions can be exchanged in our equations without affecting the results. Instead of saying that we are engaged in the double occupation of working out the cerebral consequences of stimuli and the behaviouristic consequences of cerebral processes, and of correlating these processes with conscious states, we may say with the interactionists that we are studying the causal chain Stimulus→Consciousness→Behaviour.

Therefore the procedure of interactionist psychology is justified, and Behaviourism needlessly denies itself the help which introspection could give. But a dualistic interactionist philosophy as a foundation for this procedure is not only unnecessary but misleading.

For it implies a break in the chain of physical causality which leaves the way open for the denial of the physical determinateness of animal behaviour, and for a declaration of the independence of the soul.

We now see that we may, with a clear conscience, introduce psychological expressions into the middle of a chain of physical causality. For we know that we can at any time replace the psychological term in such a heterogeneous equation by the cerebral process correlated with it, and so obtain two expressions, one causal, homogeneous, and Behaviouristic, and one correlative, heterogeneous, and psycho-physical. The difference between a causal connection and an invariable correlation is perhaps not ultimate ; but it will be convenient to speak of physical relations as causal, and psycho-physical relations as correlative.

CHAPTER II

THE IMPULSES OF THE ORGANISM

IN the first chapter we discussed the general relations between consciousness and that abstraction from our perceptual field which we call the external world. In this we shall consider more fully those parts of the external world which we call our nervous systems and their relations to our conscious states.

1. *The organism.*

The human organism is a system of receptors, *i.e.*, external and internal sense organs, and effectors, *i.e.*, striated and smooth muscles, connected by nerves. It may be compared to a complex electrical machine in which battery and wires correspond to the nervous system, switches to the receptors, and motors to the effectors. As motors operate when, and only when, the switches are on, so the effectors react when, and only when, the receptors are stimulated. Since the organism acts when it is stimulated, and continues to act until the stimulus is removed, it may be said to *seek quiescence* But in this teleological behaviour it resembles all other machines, and differs from them only in its greater complexity.

11. *Receptors and stimuli.*

Receptors, and the stimuli peculiar to them, may be conveniently classified in two different ways. We may distinguish primary from auxiliary receptors, or external from internal receptors, and the stimuli proper to each of these may be spoken of as primary and auxiliary stimuli, or as external and internal stimuli respectively. External primary receptors may be called injury-receptors (the noci-ceptors of Sherrington), and their stimuli *injuries.* They are ultimately responsible for reactions to external situations which are dangerous to the body. Internal primary receptors may be called need-receptors and their stimuli *needs.* They are responsible for the main periodic stimuli of the body, such as hunger and sensuality. Auxiliary receptors are not stimulated by injuries or needs, but they partially determine the reactions to such primary stimuli. External auxiliary receptors are the organs of sight, hearing, taste, smell, and touch. Internal auxiliary receptors include such organs as the receptors in the joints and muscle walls (the proprio-ceptors of Sherrington), and perhaps those of the semi-circular canals of the inner ear.

Two types of auxiliary stimulus deserve special notice and may be called respectively *threats* and *means.* These names more or less explain themselves, but the formal definition of them, since it depends upon the reactions elicited rather than the type of receptor stimulated, must wait for the discussion of reactions.

This classification of receptors and stimuli will be useful; but it is to some extent arbitrary, for there are no clear lines of demarcation between the different types.

12. *Stimuli and reactions.*

Among reactions there are also certain fundamental types which it is convenient to denote by special names.

Suppose a baby to be subjected to a primary external stimulus, or injury, such as a burn on the hand. This experiment is recommended by the text-books of psychology. Although the writers seldom confess that they have tried it, they do not hesitate to discuss its probable results. I think, however, we may legitimately assume that in the first experiment the baby might only scream and wriggle until it accidentally removed its hand. At this stage its reactions to an injury are random. But if the stimulus is often repeated, the reaction of withdrawing the hand, which terminates the stimulus, soon begins to occur promptly. We may say that the child has learnt the correct response which removes the stimulus, or, more shortly, that it has learnt the correct *removal*. At a still later stage the child withdraws its hand before it comes in contact with the flame. It not only removes an injury; it also avoids it. We may say that the child has learnt the correct avoidance mechanism, or, more shortly, that it has learnt the correct *avoidance*. All reactions which are purposeful and not merely random, are either removals or avoidances. And this holds whether they are learned, as in this example, or innate.

The child's random reactions and the definite removal were both evoked by a primary external stimulus or injury. But the avoidance occurred before the injury and was elicited by the sight of the candle-flame, that is, by an auxiliary external stimulus. Such stimuli may be called *threats*. The threat in the last example might perhaps be more accurately regarded as the sight of the candle-flame plus that of the hand in the vicinity, rather than as the sight of the candle-flame alone. It is this complex stimulus which behaves like an injury and gives the child no peace until it is removed. Thus, with a little charity, we may regard an avoidance as a special type of removal, that is, as the removal of a threat.

Only the simplest removals, or avoidances, consist of one act. Generally one or more preliminary acts have to be performed which establish certain conditions without which the final removal, or avoidance, is inappropriate. Thus if a baby is subjected to the primary internal stimulus of hunger, the sucking response is inadequate unless the auxiliary oral stimulus of the nipple is added to the primary visceral stimulus of hunger. The hungry infant at first reacts at random, until, partly by instinct and partly by chance, a significant cry is learnt which attracts the nipple. Then, to this fuller situation, it learns, not always without trial and error, the correct final removal of sucking. It will be convenient to call such preliminary reactions as the significant cry *seekings*,[1] and receptor stimuli, such as the oral stimulus of the nipple, *means*. Thus the adequate response to a need in the absence of a means

[1] These include the precurrent or anticipatory reactions of Sherrington.

is a seeking, and the adequate response to a *need* plus a means is a *final removal*.[1]

There may of course be a whole series of means which have to be sought before the final removal is adequate. The hungry child soon learns to seek in turn first the visual stimulus of its mother, then the oral stimulus of the nipple, before it begins to suck. It will therefore be sometimes convenient to distinguish *preliminary* from *final* means, and *preliminary* from *final* seekings. A final seeking is the reaction which immediately precedes a final removal, and a final means is a necessary constituent of the stimulus proper to a final removal.

These concepts should perhaps be illustrated by an example. Let

$$S_1 \rightarrow R_1 \rightarrow S_2 \rightarrow R_2 \rightarrow S_3 \rightarrow R_3$$

represent the successive stimuli and reactions of a hungry infant Then S_1 is the primary stimulus, *i e.*, hunger ; R_1 a preliminary seeking, *e.g.*, crying for the mother ; S_2 a preliminary means, *e.g.*, the visual stimulus of the mother's breasts ; R_2 the final seeking *i.e.*, seizing the breasts ; S_3 the final means, *i e.*, the oral stimulus of the nipple ; and R_3 the final removal, *i.e.*, sucking. S_1 of course persists throughout the train of reactions until it is removed by R_3. Each stimulus evokes a reaction. Each reaction brings about a new stimulus.

In this example seekings were steps in a complex removal. But they also occur as steps in a complex avoidance.

---

[1] This expression is a little more general than the term ' consumatory reaction ' of Sherrington.

121. *Inappropriate reactions.*

Any reaction which forms part of a train of responses terminating in the removal or avoidance of some need or injury may be said to be appropriate. And, since there are generally many different routes of different lengths to a given end, there are degrees of appropriateness in alternative reactions. Some reactions, however, do not facilitate the removals or avoidances they should, and they may therefore be said to be inappropriate. Of these there are two kinds which may be qualified respectively as *inadequate* and *irrelevant*.

An *inadequate reaction* is a reaction to a real need, injury, or threat, which does not help to remove it. If a hungry infant, instead of seeking his mother, merely sucks his own lips, his reaction is an *inadequate* removal. If, instead of seeking the nipple, he seeks his thumb, his reaction is an *inadequate seeking*. If a child, instead of jumping out of the way of a coming motor, remains frozen to the spot, like a rabbit trying to escape attention, his reaction is an *inadequate* avoidance.

An *irrelevant reaction*, on the other hand, occurs when there is no real need, injury or threat. It is a reaction to something which irrelevantly resembles a real threat. Thus, if a child who has once been burnt avoids electric light bulbs because of their irrelevant resemblance to candle flames, his reaction is an irrelevant avoidance. The stimulus which evokes such a reaction may be called a *false threat*.

All irrelevant reactions are avoidances. But seekings and removals may form part of such avoidances.

Thus loneliness to an infant may be a false threat of hunger which sets off the seeking appropriate to the real need. The lonely child calls for its mother as if it were hungry. It may even accept nourishment which it does not want when it is stimulated by such a false threat of hunger. Similarly, a fear of impotence may be a motive for excessive copulation in the absence of a real sexual need.

Perhaps the psycho-analytic theory of neurosis could be reduced to a theory of inadequate and irrelevant reactions. Such a reduction, if it were successful, might be compared with the reduction of the old fluid theory of heat to the newer kinetic theory.

2. *Cerebral processes and consciousness.*

In the first chapter we argued that the proper business of psychology was to investigate at once the causal chain ' stimulus→cerebral process→reaction ' and the correlation ' cerebral process→consciousness '. So far we have discussed certain types of stimuli and reactions, so that it remains for us to say something about the cerebral processes that form the intermediary links between them, and about the states of consciousness which are correlated with these processes.

If our knowledge of the physical side of psychology were complete, a knowledge of the cerebral disposition or engrams, left by former stimuli, would enable us to calculate what cerebral processes would follow any given stimulus. And, if psycho-physics were equally advanced, we could also determine the psychological states which would be correlated with these processes.

At present, however, a purely Behaviouristic study of a man gives us only a vague picture of the cerebral processes which mediate between his stimuli and his reactions. And this picture can only be improved by making use of an independent knowledge of the psychological states which should have been calculated from it. For, although we can neither observe cerebral processes nor calculate them from stimuli and engrams, we can compare them by assuming that similarities or differences must occur where there are similarities or differences in the observed psychological concomitants. Thus, for the present at least, cerebral physiology is of less use to introspection than introspection is to physiology.

When the baby in the imaginary experiment with the candle was exposed to the injury of a burn on its hand its reactions were at first random. If it had been able to speak it would probably have said that its consciousness contained nothing but a vague though intense feeling which we may call *pain*. And we should suppose that certain corresponding centres in the cortex (or sensorium) which we may call pain-centres, were active. If the experiment is repeated the reactions cease to be random and become definite removals. At this stage the baby would say that the pain was no longer vague, but a definite pain in the hand. And we should suppose that there was some change in the cerebral process corresponding to the changed experience and that this change had something to do with the changed response. Probably in the former case the nervous excitation from the receptors in the hand spread throughout the whole pain-centre and. thence to all the muscles of the body. Whereas, in the latter case, it passed straight through the pain-centres, only disturbing a part of them, on its way to the flexor muscles of the arm.

The baby, in the example, does not only learn to remove injuries once they have occurred ; it learns to avoid them. The retinal stimulus of the candle-flame sets off the removal mechanism before the hand comes in contact with the flame and the removal becomes an avoidance. The consciousness of the child contains a perception of the candle-flame and a memory of the pain of the burn in the hand. And this complex may be called a *fear*.

The memory of the burn which forms part of the fear may sometimes be hallucinatory and indistinguishable from the real experience. Both must then be the correlates of identical cerebral processes in the pain centres. But this central process was in one case evoked by the primary stimulus of the burn and in the other by an overflow of energy from the visual centres. It is convenient to have two names for two identical or similar psychical states when the cerebral processes which accompany them are differently conditioned. If the cerebral process is evoked by the stimulus which first caused it, we say that the corresponding psychical experience is a *sensation*. But if it is evoked by the overflow of energy from some other central process, we say that the corresponding experience is an *image*. The pain which the baby experiences when it sees the candle is correlated with a process in the pain centre. This process, however, is stimulated, not by an injury to the hand, but by an overflow from the visual centre. Therefore the baby's fear consists of the visual *sensation* of the candle flame plus an *image* of the injury.

Since the retinal impression of the candle-flame before the visual centres became associated with the pain centres would not have occasioned any marked response we must suppose that there is the same sort of difference between pain centres and visual centres as there is between primary and auxiliary receptors. It will therefore be convenient to distinguish *primary* from *auxiliary centres* and *primary* from *auxiliary cerebral processes*. In general we may say that an avoidance occurs when an auxiliary cerebral process alone stimulates the primary cerebral process whose habitual concomitant it was. Such a nervous process may be represented diagrammatically as follows :

$$P c \longrightarrow R r$$
$$A s \longrightarrow A c$$

Here A s stands for the retinal auxiliary stimulus of the candle-flame, A c for the auxiliary central process in the visual area of the cortex, P c for the primary central process in the pain centre, and R r for the removal or avoidance. The fear of the candle, which is made up of the sensation of the candle-flame plus the image of the injury, is the psychical correlate of A c + P c.

Suppose that, instead of a candle-flame, A s represented the appearance of a lion, and that the child remained rooted to the spot, petrified by fear. If the child thereby escaped the notice of the lion, its reaction would also be an adequate avoidance. But if A s represented the appearance of an approaching motor, this immobility would be an example of an inadequate avoidance.

If, however, A s represented an electric light bulb, which irrelevantly resembled a candle-flame, the reaction would have been an example of an irrelevant avoidance.

A need, like an injury, may at first stimulate only random reactions. The first time a child is subject to the need of hunger, its reactions seem to be largely random. And if it could speak it would probably say that it experienced a vague but intense discomfort which, to distinguish it from pain, we may call *want*. Presumably there is a want-centre which is stimulated by the hunger and which in turn evokes the random response. Soon, however, the child learns to suck when it is subject to the combined stimulus of hunger plus the means to its removal. And I suspect that it would say that it no longer felt a vague discomfort, but a specific appetite. The need stimulus no longer excites the whole of the want-centre, but flows straight through to the sucking reaction, only stimulating that part of the centre which is correlated with the specific want of hunger. At the same time the oral stimulus of the nipple excites its appropriate tactual centre, which in its turn augments the sucking reaction. The consciousness of the child includes the psychical correlates of both these central processes, that is, it contains a sensation of need plus a sensation of a means. It is the sum of these two kinds of

sensation that we may call an *appetite*. The whole
process may be represented diagramatically as follows :

$$P\,s \longrightarrow P\,c$$
$$\longrightarrow R\,r$$
$$A\,s \longrightarrow A\,c$$

where P s stands for the primary stimulus of hunger,
P c for the primary central process in the hunger centre,
A s for the oral auxiliary stimulus of the nipple, A c
for the auxiliary central process in the oral centre,
and R r for the removal reaction of sucking. The
appetite is the conscious correlate of P c + A c, that
is, it consists of the sensation of the need plus the
sensation of the means.

The reaction of sucking is only adequate if the nipple
is placed in the child's mouth. But as soon as it has
learnt this removal, it may at first suck whenever it is
hungry, whether the nipple is there or not. For, since
the oral means-centres[1] were in the past always activated
at some time during the continuation of processes in
the hunger want-centres, it is likely that activity in
the one excites activity in the other. Hence the
stimulus of the need alone probably flows to the need
centres and from there to the oral centres which were
formerly stimulated by the means, and these two
probably combine to discharge into the removal
mechanism of sucking. This process may be represented
diagramatically as follows :

$$P\,s \longrightarrow P\,c$$
$$\longrightarrow R\,r$$
$$A\,c$$

---

[1] An oral means-centre may be defined as a centre activity
which is correlated with the sensation, or image, of an oral means.

The psychical correlate of the two central processes is the sensation of the need plus the idea of the means. The final removal is inadequate, since it takes place in the absence of the means, and the idea of the means is hallucinatory. Such inadequate removals operate on Freud's Pleasure Principle, that is, an hallucinatory gratification takes the place of a seeking which is adequate to the realities of the situation.

Inadequate removals do not, however, remove needs, so that the child soon falls back upon random reactions until the significant cry which brings the nipple has been learnt. Thus the inadequate removal gives place to the adequate seeking, a process which may be represented as follows :

$$P\,s \longrightarrow P\,c$$
$$\longrightarrow S\,r$$
$$A\,c$$

Here, as in the last example, the conscious correlate of the cerebral process is a sensation of a need plus an image of a means. But the idea is no longer an hallucination. We must suppose that there is some difference in the central process in the two cases ; for there is some difference, other than in their results, between an ordinary idea and an hallucination.

The combination of the sensation of a need plus the idea of a means may be called a *desire*. A desire thus differs from an appetite. This was defined as the sensation of a need plus the sensation of a means.

There is a difference between the rather painful and anxious longing for an imagined means which is not yet attained and the pleasurable anticipations of the immediate removal of the need when the means is already before us. It seems legitimate to reserve the words desire and appetite for these two states. Thus, when we are hungry and imagine food, we may be said to experience desire ; but when the food is already before us, that is, when the visual image of the means has become a visual sensation, we may say that the desire has become an appetite. Sensations arising from salivary and other anticipatory reactions are, of course, more evident in appetite than in desire, but the above definition does not include their presence or absence as a criterion.

After the cerebral correlate of the desire has evoked the appropriate seeking Sr, the means appears and the stimuli complex changes from Ps to $Ps + As$. The adequate response to this situation has already been learnt, and the addition of As to Ps, and the more active disturbance of Ac which this entails are probably sufficient to cause a reversion to it.

Just as there are threats of injuries that set off appropriate removals before the injury occurs, so there are also threats of needs that evoke seekings before the need arises. Loneliness seems to excite such avoidances in children. But, since the lonely child is not really deserted, loneliness is a false threat of hunger, and his cries are irrelevant avoidances.

Sometimes a means alone, in the almost complete absence of a real need, may set off a removal. We all know, for instance, that certain culinary sights or odours may produce a fictitious appetite, even when we are not hungry, and that other visual or tactual sensa are followed by that erotic excitement which is the sexual equivalent of appetite. In such cases the activity in the auxiliary centres correlated with the sensation of the means seems to excite the need centre with which it was formerly associated. Thus, such fictitious appetites consist of the idea of a need plus the sensation of a means. The presence of the means seems to operate as a false threat of the need.

Perhaps fictitious appetites do not occur in the complete absence of a need, for we know that there are moments when the most savoury dish, or the most seductive situation, are without their appeal. But it is at least true that a means has the property of apparently increasing a need by stimulating the corresponding want-centre. An erotic situation, whether tactual or visual, is an especially important example of such a means.

Removals evoked by fictitious appetites, *i.e.* by means alone, are irrelevant.

Although irrelevant avoidances of all kinds do not remove or avoid real injuries or needs, they may nevertheless remove false threats. Psychologically, the anxiety evoked by a false threat may be as painful as that evoked by a real one. The irrelevant avoidance which removes it has therefore a psychic adequacy. Thus, for example, the lonely child finds a psychologically real consolation when it sucks its thumb, for the false threat of hunger is thereby relieved.

As a further complication we may note that a false threat may bring about a real primary stimulus. For example, it may cause the secretion of large quantities of adrenalin. The reaction which terminates or removes this stimulus is therefore in one sense adequate. But it is also in another sense irrelevant, because it is part of a train of responses evoked by a false threat.

Many neurotic symptoms and even sublimations are of this irrelevant nature. They remove, or seek to remove, superfluous anxieties which have been brought about by false threats. But there are also symptoms and sublimations which are inadequate reactions to real needs. They persist because the adequate reaction is inhibited by an irrelevant avoidance.

The connections between stimuli, cerebral processes, and reactions, together with the conscious correlates, which we have so far considered, may be conveniently tabulated as follows :

Stimulus	Cerebral process (and conscious correlate)	Reaction
Injury	Total pain centre (vague intense pain = indefinite sensation of injury)	Inadequate removal (i.e. random reactions)
Injury	Local pain centre (localised pain = definite sensation of injury)	Removal (e.g. withdrawal of hand)
Threat	Local pain centre + auxiliary centre (fear = sensation of threat + idea of injury)	Avoidance[1]

[1] If the threat is real, the avoidance may be adequate or inadequate ; if it is false, the avoidance is irrelevant.

Stimulus	Cerebral process (and conscious correlate)	Reaction
Need	Total want centre (vague intense want = indefinite sensation of need)	Inadequate removal (i.e. random reactions)
Need + Means	Local want centre + Auxiliary centre (appetite = sensation of need + means)	Removal (e.g. sucking)
Need alone	Local want centre + Auxiliary centre (sensation of need + hallucination of means)	Inadequate removal (e.g. sucking in absence of nipple)
Need alone	Local want centre + Auxiliary centre (desire = sensation of need + idea of means)	Adequate seeking (e.g. the significant cry, or grasping the nipple)
Absence of means (false threat of need)	Local want centre + Auxiliary centre (neurotic desire = idea of need + idea of means)	Irrelevant seeking (part of an irrelevant avoidance e.g. of hunger)
Means alone (false threat of need)	Local want centre + Auxiliary centre (fictitious appetite = idea of need + sensation of means)	Irrelevant removal (part of an irrelevant avoidance e.g. of hunger)

To a superficial introspection, the seeking of certain situations that we like seems more fundamental than the removal or avoidance of situations that we do not like. And, as long as this point of view is held, there can be no correlation of psychology with Behaviourism. The discussion of the last two sections may facilitate a juster sense of proportion and a realisation that nothing is ever sought which is not a *means* (adequate or inadequate) to the *removal* or *avoidance* of a real or false injury or need.

3. *Instinct and intelligence.*

The subject of this book is the development of the sexual impulses ; but we have not yet defined this term, and it is time that we remedied the omission. The term may be used either in a psychological or in a physiological sense. In the psychological sense it evidently denotes a want, desire, or appetite. Therefore, in the physiological sense it must stand for the cerebral process correlated with any of these. In practice, however, so little is known of such cerebral processes that it is necessary to refer to them in terms of the reactions which tend to follow them. I shall use the word impulse indiscriminately both in the psychological and in the physiological sense. In the last sections we have considered certain impulses, their dependence upon stimuli, and their determination of reactions.

The impulses of our biological ancestors were different from ours, and the impulses of children are different from those of grown-up people. Thus impulses may be said to develop. They may be developed either by the race or by the individual. An impulse developed by the race is said to be *innate* or the result of instinct, but if it is developed by the individual it is said to be *acquired* or the result of *intelligence.*

Impulses are determined by the structure of the nervous matter in which they occur (*e.g.*, the relative

synaptic resistence between different neurones). And
the nervous structure may be determined by heredity
alone, or partly by heredity and partly by intelligence.
Sometimes an innate impulse may remain dormant
for a part of the life of the organism. The nervous
structure is there, but it is not stimulated. Thus, the
nervous structure which determines the form of the
sexual impulse is probably to a great extent perfect
even in the child, though the glands which stimulate
the sexual need are not developed, so that the sexual
need centres are not fully stimulated. When later
the need occurs, it stimulates the sexual impulse, and
this is probably not merely a vague want, but a fairly
definite desire. Thus, since a desire includes the idea
of a means, it is probable that ideas are to some extent
innate.

An acquired impulse is determined by an acquired
nervous structure. In the higher animals every
nervous process appears to alter the resistance of
synapses, and so changes the nervous structure. Thus,
higher organisms react differently to the same situation
at different times. The original nervous structure
must always be innate. Consequently, an acquired impulse is always the modification of an innate
impulse.

In some organisms, such as insects, the nervous
structure is not very plastic, so that their impulses
are only slightly modifiable. In other words, they
act by instinct rather than by intelligence. In man
the nervous structure is more plastic than in any
other animal. He acts more by intelligence than by

instinct. Even the act of sucking, which appears to be quite instinctive in all other mammals, has to be partly learnt by a human child. It may take some time before he learns what to do with the nipple when it is placed in his mouth. But the young pig seems to have a much clearer idea of what he desires even before he has seen his mother.

3111. *Types of innate impulses.*

Innate impulses may be conveniently classified according to the degree of foresight they display or simulate. First, there are *innate impulses to final removals* evoked by the combined stimuli of a need plus the corresponding final means. Though the baby, unlike the young pig, does not seem to be able to find its own way to its mother's breasts, it may suck correctly by instinct the first time the nipple is put in its mouth, and it certainly learns to suck more quickly than it would if it had to rely solely on the selection of fortuitous random reactions. Thus the final means, *i.e.*, the oral stimulus of the nipple, together with the need, *i.e.*, hunger, innately elicits the appropriate response. The impulse to masturbate which very young children display, and to which psycho-analysts attach so great an importance, is probably another innate impulse of this kind evoked by a need plus a final means, that is, by the combined stimuli of a sexual need plus an accidental friction between the hand and the genital organ.

Next in complexity to these simple impulses come *impulses to seekings of final means* evoked by the combined stimuli of a need plus a preliminary means. The new-born pig seeks and finds its mother's teats by smell. Thus, the nasal stimulus, or preliminary means, plus the hunger, evokes a seeking of the oral stimulus of the teats, or final means. But children display such impulses less certainly than animals.

Finally there are *impulses* to *preliminary seekings* evoked by a need alone. The cry of the infant which attracts the mother is probably of this nature, but it is not followed by a definite train of precise reactions. Many of the lower animals, on the other hand, are born with impulses to whole chains of astonishingly accurate reactions, which simulate, if they do not include, great foresight. The nesting habits of birds and the migration of many animals are oft-quoted examples of reactions determined by unlearned innate impulses of this nature.

It is often assumed that such impulses do not include ideas of the final means that they seek, but at most ideas of the next stage in the process of seeking. But there is, after all, nothing supernatural in the inheritance of ideas, since this would be only the psychical correlate of the inheritance of nervous structure. Certainly the bird inherits something more than a vague want which would only evoke random reactions until the correct chain of responses was learnt by chance. And once we admit that it inherits desires, that is, wants plus ideas of means, it is as easy to suppose that the desire is general and far-sighted as that it is specific and confined to the next step. It seems in fact easier to suppose that the bird inherits a general desire to

D

build a nest than a specific desire to join sticks together.[1]

3112. *The imperfection of innate impulses.*

In general the higher the organism the less precise and perfect are its innate impulses. This lack of precision characterises both the response and the stimulus which evokes it. The perfected response is a learned modification of the crude innate response, the imperfection of which is but the necessary condition of adaptability. And the relevant stimulus is a selection from a class of stimuli patterns many of which are false. Thus, the new-born infant often blows and splutters before it sucks correctly, and the new-born chick pecks at nasty grubs which inadequately resemble the grain it likes.

A stimulus which irrelevantly evokes a response relevant to another stimulus, or which is sought because of an inadequate resemblance to a real means, may be said to be a symbol. A symbol in the restricted psycho-analytic sense is probably an irrelevant stimulus to an innate impulse which resembles some means or threat. Convex and concave objects, we know, are found to be universal phallic and vagina symbols. In other words, they excite some of the innate impulses which are relevant to these objects. Perhaps it is largely because the human child is prevented from perfecting his instincts by imitation and experiment that he reacts to so many symbols. When an avoidance has been superimposed upon a seeking, the symbol may become a false threat and the object of a phobia.

[1] Cf. Chapter III, 21.

Thus, the snake phobia of the young woman is often an avoidance superimposed upon a seeking, which would be relevant to the object symbolised but which is irrelevant to the symbol.

312. *Types of acquired impulse.*

Acquired impulses also may be divided into two types ; those which are imitated and those which are invented. Those which a man acquires by imitation or instruction compose the cultural tradition of his species, and may be called *cultural impulses* ; while those which he has invented form his more private contribution to his psychology and may be called *private impulses.*

The division of impulses into innate and acquired, and of acquired impulses into cultural and private, is useful but artificial. It would be more exact to say that the impulses of man are the result of three factors—inherited nervous structure, tradition, and originality—than that they are of three types—innate, cultural, and private. The impulses of insects are mainly one-dimensional and determined by inherited structure alone, those of primitive man are mainly two-dimensional and determined by innate structure plus tradition, and those of modern man are three-dimensional and determined by innate structure, tradition, and invention.

According to Marais' observations[1], baboons do not develop appropriate sexual impulses unless instinct is assisted by the example of the older generation.

[1] *Psyche*, October, 1926.

Possibly many of the perversions to which the human race is subject, may be due, not solely to inhibitions, but also to a lack of positive instruction. At least the converse is true. Malinowski's Trobrianders, who were exposed from earliest infancy to the influence of the sexual example of their elders, do not develop perversions.[1]

3121. *Theories of instinct* : *Darwin and Lamarck.*

Every European now believes in evolution and that all forms of life are descended from one simple form. But there are two views of the method by which the great variations have been brought about.

According to one view, which may be called the Darwinian theory, although it is an exaggeration of what Darwin himself believed, the nature of the germ cell determines the nature of the body, or soma, which protects it, but the dependence is not reciprocal, so that evolution can proceed by the variation of the germ cell alone. Such variation may be due to two causes. It may result either from conjugation with another cell which introduces a new factor, or from a spontaneous mutation. The laws of variation by crossing, first investigated by Mendel, can only account for the relative frequency of different permutations of *existing* factors, and cannot explain the whole of evolution. But, by a finite number of finite *spontaneous* variations, however small, mutations in the germ cell sufficient to determine any degree of variation in its protecting body may be achieved—though for great

[1] *The Sexual Life of Savages*, 44 sq., 395 sq.).

changes a vast number of steps are naturally required.

According to the other theory of evolution, which is called the Lamarckian theory, there is a reciprocal reaction between the germ cell and the soma, so that evolution proceeds both by the spontaneous and the Mendelian variation of the germ cell and the modifications produced in it by the characters which the soma has acquired in its individual life. Thus the Lamarckian theory requires fewer steps to achieve a given change. But, since the germ plasm appears to be isolated from the soma from a very early age, it is almost impossible to imagine any mechanism by which it could be influenced at all precisely by changes in the soma. How, for instance, can we suppose that those minute changes in cerebral structure, which are correlated with acquired intelligence, evoke those precise changes in the germ cells which determine similar cerebral modifications in the offspring? For these reasons, and because of the absence of conclusive evidence in its favour, the Lamarckian theory is generally discredited. It is not yet, however, definitely disproved.[1]

It is to be feared that at present political rather than scientific motives often determine an allegiance to either theory. Thus the parental jealousy of the educated plebeian will incline him to the theory of

[1] Some psycho-analysts have argued that the presence of certain complexes can only be explained along Lamarckian lines. But if they had been alive to the immense physiological difficulty of accepting this view they would probably not have abandoned so soon the attempt to discover an alternative solution of their problem.

Lamarck, while that of the unlettered patrician will bias him in favour of the Darwinian view.

Common to both theories is an explanation of the absence of theoretically possible types. The individual who does not protect his germ cells, either when they are within his body through failing to protect himself, when they leave his body through failing to deposit them where they can grow a new body, or when they are outside it through failing to protect his young, will leave no progeny to perpetuate his racial immorality. Thus, of the innumerable types which might have existed, only those whose self-preservative, reproductive, and maternal impulses are well developed, and who have in consequence best cared for the germ cells which have been handed down to them, have survived until this day.

32. *A theory of intelligence.*

It is a fundamental assumption of this book that animal behaviour can ultimately be explained by chemistry and physics. We are of course still a long way from this achievement, but we are already in a position to guess at the sort of mechanisms which determine what reaction will follow a given stimuli complex, and how these mechanisms are modified in educable animals to form acquired reactions better adapted to their needs.

The unit of the nervous system is the neurone, which usually consists of a nucleus, some short branches, or dendrites, and one long branch or axon. Each neurone contains stored potential energy which, when released by a stimulus to a dendrite, sets up a wave of chemical decomposition along the axon. Such a discharge appears to dissipate the potential energy of the neurone, so that it requires a certain period to recover between each wave. This period is called the refractory period. If the intervals between stimuli are shorter than the refractory period, the neurone will be fatigued and will transmit no waves of disturbance.

The point of contact of the axon, or efferent process, of one cell and a dendrite, or afferent process, of another is called a synapse. We may represent the nervous system as a complex network in which the knots are the synapses, and the string between them, the neurones. As each knot is the meeting place of several strings, so each neurone is capable of being stimulated by several cells, and of transmitting its energy to several others.

Whether or not a particular cell b will be stimulated by some other cell a with which it is in contact must depend upon two factors, the excitability of the cell itself and the resistance of the synapse. If b is already being stimulated by a third neurone a' and the waves of excitation from a fall in its refractory period, it will be completely fatigued and unable to transmit the stimulus. And the same effect will result if the resistance of the synapse is too high to permit the passage of the stimulus. If, however, the stimuli from a' and a arrive in phase, it seems likely that they will more easily break through the synaptic resistance.[1]

It is further supposed that the resistance of a synapse

[1] See Keith Lucas, *The Conduction of the Nervous Impulse.*

is reduced during a succession of waves of nervous disturbance and that it does not completely recover. Hence the resistance is lessened after each occasion on which it has been broken down. It will perhaps be worth while to see how far these known and assumed properties of the nervous system can account for animal behaviour.

321 *The acquisition of simple removals.*

Watson has suggested that simple removals, such as the reaction of a child to a burn on the hand, are learnt as habits because they happen more often than any other response.[1] The correct response must always happen before the stimulus is removed. Thus the correct response must happen as often as the stimulus, whereas other random reactions need not always occur. It is therefore likely that after many repetitions of a given injury the correct removal will have occurred more often than any other. And, if the synaptic boundary between neurones loses some of its resistance each time a nervous discharge passes it, a given neural path becomes more probable the more it is followed. Hence the correct response, which happens most often, will become the most probable, and the organism will profit by experience.

It has been objected to this explanation that learning does not take place gradually, but in jerks, and that introspection can detect the exact moment at which the correct response is learnt. But the phenomena which are disclosed by introspection seem to be the

[1] *Psychology from the Standpoint of a Behaviorist,* 1919, p. 294.

phenomena of recognition, in which an old response is suddenly found to be appropriate, with slight modifications, to a new situation. Such recognition depends upon the previous existence of other learned reactions, and although these in turn may be super-imposed upon others to form a hierarchy from the simple to the complex, there must ultimately be simple learned reactions which cannot be formed by the modification of others more simple, and which must therefore be formed in some way such as Watson suggests.

322. *The acquisition of simple avoidances.*

The acquisition of avoidances also can be plausibly explained by mechanical parallels. It was argued in a former section that such reactions must depend upon the stimulation of primary centres from auxiliary centres (though in some cases the whole process may be purely spinal). Thus, when the child avoids the threat of the candle-flame, the central processes in the visual centres, which are correlated with the sight of the candle, must stimulate the pain centres ; and these in turn must evoke the removal which has already been learnt as the correct response to the injury of the burn. A suggested explanation for this stimulation of a primary centre from an auxiliary centre, which produces the avoidance of injuries before they occur, has been given by many psychologists. It has been pointed out that, if the resistance of the synapses to the passage of a nervous discharge decreases during a discharge, an auxiliary stimulus which happened often to occur at the same time as some primary stimulus would flow into the same common path, and so wear for itself a channel which would ensure that it would in future alone evoke the response appropriate to the primary stimulus. Thus we may suppose that the retinal impression of the candle-flame, or threat, which is the invariable concomitant of the primary stimulus of the burn, after stimulating the visual centres, flows over into the pain centres, which were originally stimulated by the burn, and so evokes the same.response.

323. *The acquisition of seekings.*

The central processes which evoke seekings seem more complex than those which evoke simple removals and avoidances. It is at first difficult to see how the organism can progress from the inadequate removal in the absence of a means to the appropriate seeking. Why should not the removal (*e.g.*, the sucking), which is learned as the adequate response to a need (*e.g.*, hunger) in the presence of a means (*e.g.*, the oral stimulus of the nipple), persist indefinitely as an inadequate removal in the absence of the means? I suppose that the answer to this question is that the neurones which are active during the inadequate removal are eventually fatigued, so that the primary stimulus, which still persists, discharges in different directions, producing new random reactions, until the correct seeking (*e.g.*, the significant cry) is learnt.

324. *The acquisition of inhibitions.*

If our theory of avoidance is correct, an avoidance is a premature removal which occurs before the primary stimulus, to which the removal is appropriate, and so prevents the stimulus from ever taking place. But sometimes an avoidance is superimposed upon a previous seeking, as, for instance, when a child first tends to grasp all bright objects and then to avoid all those that cause him pain. In such cases, though the two reactions at first succeed each other, as when the child draws back from the candle-flame which he has started to grasp, the double reaction soon changes into no reaction at all. The seeking is not cut short by an avoidance ; it is inhibited. Now an inhibition is not a reaction, like an avoidance, but a nervous process which actively prevents a reaction. How does it develop ?

The central processes which evoke avoidances undoubtedly acquire the property of simply inhibiting the antagonistic seeking. But this property is really not peculiar to such processes ; it is common to all impulses, for no reaction can take place unless all antagonistic reactions are inhibited. Thus every reaction is accompanied by a number of inhibitions, or, in other words, the nervous impulse which evokes a given reaction has both a positive and a negative side ; it evokes the reaction and inhibits its rivals.

We have seen that a neurone may be fatigued into inactivity by a periodic stimulus the period of which is shorter than its own refractory period, and that this condition may occur if the neurone is stimulated from two or more separate sources which are out of phase. Hence an inhibition is perhaps a nervous process which bombards a neurone with stimuli out of phase with the stimuli which it is already receiving. Whether or not the activity of a central process C will facilitate or inhibit the effects of a central process C' in evoking a given motor neurone will depend upon whether or not the neural waves from C and C' are in phase. This will probably depend upon the relative lengths of the paths taken from C and C' to the motor neurone. A facilitating discharge will take a path of such a length that it will arrive in phase with discharges from C', and an inhibiting discharge will take a path of such a length that it will arrive out of phase.

We know that a stimulus persists until the appropriate reaction which removes it, occurs, and that, for this reason, the appropriate reaction tends to occur more often than any inappropriate alternative. We have just seen that the nervous impulse which evokes such an appropriate reaction has a negative, as well as a positive, side. The appropriate inhibiting impulses must occur as often as the appropriate facilitating impulses. They also must, therefore, tend to occur more often than any inappropriate alternative and to wear for themselves a neural path of least resistance. Hence the inhibition of antagonistic reactions may be learnt at the same time and in the same way as the impulses which evoke a removal.

Psychologists sometimes speak of tension dammed up by inhibitions which must find some other outlet. But from the neurological point of view it would seem that increase of tension is only indirectly due to inhibitions. There is no reason to suppose that the tension in a neurone is greater after it has failed to excite another neurone than after it has been successful. For the nervous process is not a wave of pressure of a fluid in a pipe, but a wave of chemical decomposition ; and a fuse, which is a truer analogy, does not burn brighter if it fails to explode the mine. If, however, an inhibition prevents the removal or avoidance of some injury, need, or threat, the stimulus remains or increases. In this sense alone can inhibitions increase tension. Thus analogies from hydrodynamics, although useful, may be misleading, and should be applied with caution. They were introduced into psychology by Descartes, and are still sometimes used by those who, in professing to distrust neurology, limit themselves to the neurological parallels of a bygone age.

CHAPTER III

THE PHYLOGENESIS OF IMPULSES

IN the last chapter we distinguished certain fundamental types of impulse and discussed the general theory of their development. In this and in the following two chapters we shall be concerned with the development of specific impulses in the race, in culture, and in the individual.

The phylogeny of impulses, or the racial history of their evolution, is the history of the evolution of innate impulses in so far as these can be abstracted from the influence of the cultural and individual environment. The cultural history of impulses is the history of the growth of custom, while the ontogeny of impulses includes an account of the successive appearance of innate impulses in the individual, as well as of how he acquires the culture of his species, and of how he makes his individual contribution to his own psychology.

In this chapter I shall try to review some of the steps through which the various adequate reactions to the needs of man, and his corresponding desires and appetites, have been evolved. Such an attempt is necessarily both speculative and incomplete. At best it can only indicate the main outline of the kind of systematic presentation of instinctual development which seems to me desirable.

1. *The biology of instincts.*

The psychologist who is concerned with the evolution of impulses should always remember that the biologist has already laid the foundations of his science. If he neglects to bear this fact constantly in mind his imposing speculations, however alluring and consistent they may be in themselves, may collapse before the first blast of serious criticism. This is my excuse for prefacing the discussion of the obscurer impulses, with which we are primarily concerned, by a summary of what the biologist, as I understand him, tells us of the fundamental stages in evolution.

11. *Division.*

The series from the chemically simple to the biologically complex proceeds by even steps, so that one must define arbitrarily the point where life began. We may start, however, with one of the protozoa from which we are all derived, and attempt to follow its biography. Such a protozoon already possessed a stable structure which persisted during the interchange of atoms between it and its environment. But it did not only persist ; it also grew, until the structure became unstable and split into two cells almost exactly alike. These cells grew and divided in their turn, and so on for countless generations. Now although the two parts into which these cells split were nearly alike, we must suppose that there was some difference.

Some property which the parent possessed was accentuated in one of its offspring and diminished in the other, so that each resembled its parent more closely than its sister. Since this process of deviation was continued in all generations, great differences finally developed.

Of all these possible mutations of the original cell which might in time have been produced by successive division, some would have been better adapted to their environment than others. But in each generation the less adapted tended to perish rather than to transmit their structural character to two descendants. Thus the later generations were a selection from many possible types

To this stage of evolution, since there is no difference between germ plasm and soma, the Darwinian and Lamarckian theories equally apply.

12. *Conjugation.*

The cells grew by devouring their environment and building it into their own structure. Sometimes also they must have devoured other cells like themselves and so saved the energy necessary to change the molecular structure of their diet. In certain species it became a condition of growth and life that cells should sometimes devour each other, that is, that they should sometimes reunite.

In some such way as this, the conjugation of protozoan cells may have originated. But whatever its origin many species became unable to live and divide unceasingly unless this process of division was from time to time interrupted by the opposite process of reunion. Such species evolved more rapidly than their parthenogenetic neighbours, because each individual inherited mutations not only from one but from several lines of ancestors.

13. *Differentiation*.

131. *Differentiation of cells into germ plasm and soma*.

In certain species the cells did not always separate when they divided, but remained as united though distinct individuals. The outer ones were then specialized as a protective covering, lost the power of conjugation, and so, perhaps, become mortal. But the inner cells, or germ plasm, retained their original character, and from time to time conjugated with other like cells and grew about them a new body.

132. *Differentiation of germ cells into male and female*.

If germ cells within the body conjugated only with each other, the purpose of conjugation, which seems to have been rapidly to diffuse mutations, would have been largely lost. Hence Nature evolved a cellular exogamy.[1] The germ cells were specialized into two kinds, male and female, which could only conjugate with each other.

133. *Differentiation of soma into male and female*.

At first both male and female germ cells developed in different compartments of the same body. But perhaps to secure a completer cellular exogamy the soma also was differentiated into two types, one con-

---

[1] *i.e.* She favoured those which happened to be exogamous.

E

taining only the male germ cells and the other only the female.

134. *Variation and selection of soma.*

With the development of soma a different type of character became of survival value to the germ plasm. In the protozoa it is only the vitality of the germ cell itself which is important. But in the germ cells of the metazoa the disposition to the formation of specific bodies is the chief factor in survival. Those cells which grew inefficient bodies perished. But those whose bodies were adapted to their environment perpetuated their body-forming characters with slight modifications, of which the least adapted were again eliminated and the most efficient selected. Thus in course of time great changes were effected, and bodies developed which protected themselves as long as they contained the germ cells, and which discharged these cells from time to time in an environment where they were most likely to combine with other cells of the right kind. They possessed these characters because, of all variations which had yet occurred, they best secured the continued existence of the germ cells. If they had not possessed these characters, they would not have survived. Thus it was the elimination by nature of unadapted types rather than the guiding hand of Providence that gave the appearance of a purposeful evolution. Probably the spontaneous variations of the germ cells were alone transmitted ; but Lamarckians believe that characters developed by the soma within its own life modified these cells.

14. *Internal fertilization.*

At first, the soma discharged the germ cells into the water where chance determined whether or not they would combine with other cells and grow new bodies. But variations which had gregarious tendencies during the period of breeding, and discharged their cells at the same time and place as other members of the species, secured for them more favourable opportunities for combination and growth. Hence these types throve and multiplied and other types tended to be crowded out.

The sea became over-populated. Some species developed characters which enabled them to crawl out upon the land for part of their lives and so to protect themselves. They tended to multiply, and gave rise to the race of the amphibia. But they could not live all their lives upon the earth, for the germ cells still had to be deposited in the water before they could combine and grow new bodies. Those individuals which did not return to the water died out and so failed to transmit their habits.

Variations arose, however, the males of which deposited their seed within the females, so that the cells combined within her body and not fortuitously in the water. And when variations of these variations began to live entirely upon land they did not die out, but, surrounded by much food and free from enemies, multiplied exceedingly.

Ferenczi has suggested[1] that the amphibia first learnt coitus by seeking the proximity of each other's wet

[1] *Versuch einer Genitaltheorie.*

bodies as a substitute for the sea which they had left. We know that in dreams a woman is often represented by water. I remember one small boy of two who used the same word for water as for mother. Thus if a woman is still a symbol of the sea, which our amphibian ancestors sought as the means of evoking the discharge of their germ cells, coitus is, as Ferenczi suggests, a substitute for a return to the sea (thalassal regression). This suggestion is interesting and possibly correct. But it is not, as he thinks, conclusive proof of the theory of Lamarck. As Lloyd Morgan has pointed out, an acquired modification may act as a foster-nurse to a spontaneous variation in the same direction.[1] A tendency to find a substitute for the sea in the damp body of a female might well arise spontaneously, and, if it were supported by an acquired tendency in the same direction, its survival value would be increased. It would thus be likely to be fixed and improved by the elimination of variations which least possessed it. Organisms naturally seek substitutes for what they have lost. When these substitutes have an additional survival value in their own right, those variations which sought them most effectually would be selected.

15. Parturition.

Once the cells had begun to reunite within the body of the female it would be an advantage to them to enjoy

[1] Letter from Lloyd Morgan to Elliot Howard on the Survival of Coincident Variation, Elliot Howard, British Warblers, ii, summary. 20.

the protection of her body for the first period of their growth. Variations which remained longest would multiply at the expense of their more precocious brothers. In this way was evolved first the egg and finally the foetus which remains many months within its mother's womb.

Ferenczi and Rank have attempted to reduce the desire for coitus, and especially for incestuous coitus, to a desire to seek that perfect equilibrium in the womb which the child once enjoyed. The desire for coitus is thus for them a substitute for the desire to return to the womb, and in support of their hypothesis they quote dreams in which coitus is represented by birth. But the amphibia invented coitus before there was any birth, and reptiles and birds have intercourse even though they only lay eggs. Therefore the desire to return to the womb cannot be a general motive of the desire for coitus, even if it has largely economised the survival of other motives in man. It seems more likely that the tendency to return to the womb is a substitute for coitus, which is possibly itself a substitute for the tendency to return to the sea. This order would correspond more closely with the order of evolution.

16. *Lactation.*

The history of the race from the invention of birth to the present day is largely characterised by an ever-increasing dependence of the child upon its mother. At first there was a cluster of ripening cells discharged into the water, then an egg sat on or left to incubate in the sun, next a foetus protected until its birth, and finally, a child suckled by its mother. The germ cell which was first dependent upon the water for its growth became at last the child parasitic upon its mother, not only before its birth, but even for many months or years after it is born.

Ferenczi has also sought the origin of the mammal in the tendency to return to the womb. The tooth is a common symbol of the penis, and Ferenczi supposes that the child's tendency to bite its way back into the warm and comfortable place from which it so reluctantly emerged, since it had the secondary advantage of providing nourishment, was fixed and developed into the tendency to suck the teats. If so, the mammalian habit, like a sublimation, was originally an inadequate response to one need which survived because it happened to fulfil another. But it is more likely that this tendency was developed from a general carnivorous impulse which gave advantage to those species in which it was most displayed by the young and most tolerated by their mothers. In this way it might have been fixed and specialized by selection.

17. *The biography of a germ cell.*

The germ cells which we carry in our bodies are as old as life itself. They have lived for millions of years and have grown about them a series of temporary moving habitations, of which the last members are ourselves. We are excrescences about our germ cells which they have evolved to protect themselves. We are born subject to certain injuries and endowed with certain needs which we remove or avoid when we protect, feed, or reproduce ourselves, or when we protect our children. The reactions which we employ to remove or to avoid these injuries and needs are partly predetermined by the nervous structure which we have inherited. If we were not subject to these injuries and did not possess these needs, and if we were not endowed with tendencies to remove or avoid them in specific ways, we should not have existed. For our ancestors, afflicted with the same defects, would not have left offspring.

Our private purpose is to remove and avoid our needs and injuries as effectively as possible, but only if we do so in the same manner as our ancestors, shall we in turn perpetuate our race. There is thus the possibility of an opposition between the interest of the individual and that of the race. If, by intelligence, we discover more rapid methods of removing and avoiding our needs and injuries than the methods inherited as instincts, we shall presumably adopt them. But there is no guarantee that these methods will be of equal service to the race. It is possible that the most economic way of removing and avoiding injuries and needs is to seek death rather than life, and that nothing but an inherited false idea of death as a state of pain and want has prevented our race from exterminating itself. If so, we owe our existence to a series of false threats, and we shall decree our doom as soon as we discover that we have been duped. A race of automatic ants with instincts but no intelligence will live and suffer in our place.[1]

[1] *Cf.* Chapter vi, 3.

2. *The psychology of instincts.*

To each of the reactions of living organisms, which we have passed so rapidly in review, there is very possibly a psychic counterpart. There are certainly mental correlates to the later and more complex modes of instinctive behaviour of the higher animals. And, since there is no sudden break in the scale of ascending complexity of structure and function, there seems no good reason why there should be any place where the correlated consciousness begins. Therefore, we may perhaps with Leibnitz attribute some *petite perception* to the simplest function. Even the protozoon may feel distinct qualities of discomfort which impel it at one time to divide, at another to absorb nourishment, and at another to wander restlessly until it has conjugated with its mate. But its consciousness is probably limited to sensations of needs and injuries, and it is unlikely that it ever knows the joys of appetite or the miseries of desire and fear.

21. *Instinctive desires and fears.*

There is, however, little doubt that both desire and fear occur as innate impulses very low in the scale of life. If so, there must be innate ideas, for fear involves the idea of an approaching injury, and desire anticipates the sensation of a means.[1] But it is important to realize that the mere correct response to a situation the first time it is presented does not necessarily involve an innate idea. Only where such a situation, if it is a need, evokes an idea of the requisite means, or, if

[1] *Cf.* Chap. ii, 3111.

it is a threat, an idea of the coming injury, are we entitled to say that there is an innate idea.

It is, however, hard to believe that instinctive reactions which are well adapted and highly specialized do not involve some anticipation of what they seek or avoid. We have seen that the central process which evokes an avoidance or a seeking in a higher animal includes activity in the centres correlated with the idea or sensation of the avoided injury or sought means, as well as in the centres correlated with the idea or sensation of the threat or need.[1] It seems probable that this is a general rule. And if so, some idea of the injury avoided or the means sought must be part of the psychic correlates of all avoiding or seeking impulses.

But we need not suppose that such ideas are necessarily conscious. That part of the innate nervous structure which determines innate impulses may well be in a lower neural centre than that part of the cortex named the sensorium, activity in which is correlated with consciousness. Therefore, instinctive desires and fears perhaps exist first in the unconscious, and are later duplicated in consciousness after the means which they seek and the injuries which they avoid have been discovered or experienced. If, however, a seeking is actively inhibited, the corresponding conscious desire may never occur and its unconscious counterpart may remain unmodified by trial and error.

Most animals seem to avoid their hereditary enemies at once, even if the example of the older generation

[1] *Cf.* Chap. ii, 2.

has never taught them to do so. This reaction is more pronounced in species in which the young are left to hatch out by themselves and are not protected and educated by their parents, whereas among higher animals instinct has atrophied to make room for the more perfect adaptations which result from imitation and intelligence. But it seems certain that all species inherit innate fears of some kind, and that these include innate ideas of injuries.

It is probable that there are innate ideas of threats as well as of injuries. It is difficult to deny that the young animal recognizes its hereditary enemy the first time it sees him, when it avoids him so correctly. And this recognition would seem to imply a latent idea of the specific threat and not merely an innate association between the threat and the injury. Further, the young animal not only avoids its enemy when it sees him ; it also flies or hides when it hears his characteristic rustle or call. It seems likely that this rustle or call excites the idea of the enemy. If so, the threat of a threat may innately evoke the idea of a threat.

Similarly, all animals seem to inherit in a varying degree the capacity to recognize their proper food or mate. Even if this recognition does not involve the innate idea of the food or mate, it excites a desire which includes as one of its constituents the idea of the oral or genital sensation which is the final means. Thus, appetite, which we have defined as the sensation of a need plus the idea of the final means,[1] is likely to be

---

[1] *Cf.* Chap. ii, 2.

innate But probably we can go further than this and attribute to many animals innate seekings of whole series of preliminary means If so, the want, even the first time it occurs, may excite a dim or definite idea of the food or mate which would still the need.

22. *The sexual impulse.*

Classical biology divides innate impulses into instincts of self-preservation and reproduction. Like all classifications of an infant science this division is arbitrary. We might attempt a classification based on the discussion of stimuli and reactions in the second chapter, and divide instincts into innate avoidances and innate seekings. But in practice this division would be almost equally difficult to maintain. I have therefore attempted instead to follow up some of the contributions to, and derivatives of, a single instinct. If this were done conscientiously, it would involve a discussion of every impulse ; for there are no sharp boundaries to distinguish each from the rest. Perhaps it would be possible to begin such an investigation from any angle. But I have chosen to discuss the sexual instinct, which seems to have the furthest ramifications, and the most intimate relations with all the rest.

There has been a tendency of late years to promote the Empedoclean Eros to the position of an all-embracing urge of which every other impulse is a mode. The concept of love has in consequence become excessively confused. In its simplest form it appears to be identical with the desire for a mate, that is, it is an emotion made up of the sensation of a sexual need plus the idea of the preliminary and final means to the removal of this need ; it anticipates the visual, olfactory, and tactual presence of the mate. But it is impossible to restrict the term of love to this narrow emotion. Many impulses have contributed to make up the full experience, and it has itself contributed to many others. We may therefore consider in turn a variety of impulses in order to discover, if possible, how far each has contributed *to* sensuality and how far it is itself a derivative *from* the sexual impulse.[1]

221. The oral impulse.

Psycho-analysts have found that there is no sharp division between the infant's desire for his mother's milk and the adult's love of his wife, and they have used the same word to describe both yearnings. Among pre-mammalian animals, and especially among those which do not even bring food to their young, there can be no such easy bridge between sexual and alimentary desires. Since the two impulses appear to have been separately evolved, it would seem at first sight that it should be possible to distinguish them more clearly in man than psycho-analysts believe. But the work of the analysts cannot be so easily

---

[1] A terminology which distinguishes a plurality of impulses derived from all the fundamental needs of the organism, each of which may contribute to, or be partly derived from, a sexual impulse, seems to me more helpful than one in which every impulse is either classified as sexual or destructive or as a fusion of these two.

neglected, and, if we refuse to adopt their wider definition of love, we must restrict it far below its former scope. If we cannot call the infant's desire for food sexual, it would seem that we must also deny this quality to the desires for all those oral activities, such as kissing, which are derived from the sucking habits of the infant and precede or complicate the sexual act.[1] Perhaps the difficulty will disappear if we admit that, although nutritional and sexual impulses may be distinct in lower animals, in mammals, and especially in man, accidental variations of each impulse have been adapted to reinforce the other. We have already mentioned Ferenczi's theory of the way in which the sexual impulse may have assisted the development of the sucking habit of young mammals.[2] We have now to consider the contribution which this nutritional instinct has made to the instinct of reproduction in mammals and especially in man.

I do not know whether reptiles display oral affection for their mates, but we may fairly suppose that the main oral contribution to sexual love was made after animals began to feed, and especially to suckle their young. We may suppose, further, that the sucking impulse, once it was evolved, was liable in the individual to survive its real utility and to persist as an irrelevant removal of a false threat of hunger. Such a neurotically persistent oral desire for the mother would be readily transferable to the mate. She would thus become

---

[1] *Sie trank meiner Küsse lodernde Glut mit Dürsten und mit Lechzen*, Heine.

[2] *Cf.* § 16.

doubly valuable ; for she would be the means, not only to the removal of a real genital need, but also to the removal of a false nutritional threat.[1] And the over-developed oral desire, since it would strengthen the purely sexual ties, would possess survival value and tend to be selected. Thus, what was originally a useless prolongation into maturity of an infantile dependence would become an integral part of the sexual impulse. Before this time the mate was probably not loved as a person but desired for her sexual organs alone, and much which at the present day makes sexual love richer must be due to this secondary adaptation of desires which were originally evolved to satisfy another need.

Oral habits, such as licking, form an important element in the courting of many of the higher mammals. A dog will bite the ear and lick the face of a bitch in order to excite her. And the boar will exert himself in a similar manner when he is courting a sow. In man, where the infancy period is so much longer, one would naturally expect that the oral contribution to sexuality would be correspondingly increased.

222. The anal impulse.

The anal impulse is, of course, distinct from the sexual impulse, for it relieves a different need. But psycho-analysts have shown that each has borrowed something from the other. We may inquire exactly what is meant by this and ask whether evolution or education is the more responsible.

[1] *Cf.* Chap. ii, 121 ; Chap. v, 22.

The child, according to the observations of analysts, takes a sexual interest in the act of defecation, in the organs that perform this function, and in their products. These three interests often recur in the adult as fixed sexual perversions, or as exciting pre-liminaries to the normal sexual act. We may consider them in turn.

2221. *The act of defecation.*

The anus has evolved from a common cloaca which performed the functions of sex as well as of excretion, so that it is not biologically surprising that its stimulation should still sometimes excite erotic feelings similar to those produced by the stimulation of the male or female organs. It is well known that effeminate homosexual males not infrequently enjoy the passive stimulation of the anus, and this no doubt forms for them the only satisfaction of feminine desires which their anatomy permits. But the opposite perversion also exists, and some men, especially before puberty or after they are old and impotent, find their pleasure not in normal ejaculation but in an aggressive expulsion of their faeces. These are extreme cases, but Ferenczi has suggested[1] that even among normal people some part of the impulse to ejaculation may be derived from the impulse to defecate. For nature is economical, and has made use, as far as she can, not only of the same organs but also of the same nervous structure and corresponding innate impulses for two different purposes.

[1] *Versuch einer Genitaltheorie*

2222. The organs of defecation.

The child's interest in the organs of defecation is no doubt largely due to their association with the pleasure of their function, but it is also partly due to two other causes. There is a resemblance between the breasts and the buttocks, which facilitates the transference to the latter of an affection first developed for the former, and many psycho-analyses have proved that this transference frequently, if not always, occurs to some extent. Besides these reasons for the transference to the anal region of interest directed originally to other things, there is little doubt that this region innately excites the sexual impulse. The ancestors of man, like other animals, copulated *a tergo*, and this practice, in spite of its censure by the Roman Church, is not even yet extinct. Thus an anal tropism must have been evolved by our pre-human ancestors as a necessary preliminary to the sexual act, which has survived as an embarrassing alternative to the more direct approach.

2223. The products of defecation.

The interest in the products of defecation seems even more difficult to explain than the interest in its function or organs. The smell may have been utilized by evolution as a sexual stimulus. At least it is attractive to dogs always and to children sometimes. I knew a boy of four who was always pleasurably excited by what he called delicious nasty smells. The typical coprophilic pervert, as psycho-analysis has shown, has transferred to the products of the anus the affection which he once bore for the products of the breast. Possibly an innate olfactory tropism facilitates this transference of interest.

223. *The urethral impulse.*

Urethral perversions have long been recorded, and they appear not to be confined to man. Mares on heat, for instance, are said to urinate when they hear the stallion neigh.[1] But it has been reserved for psychoanalysts to argue that there is a urethral contribution to the normal sexual impulse.[2] There was once a common cloaca for three functions, and it is likely that the same nervous mechanism is still shared partly by all three. Infantile troubles over urination, which form a considerable part of the worries of children at a certain age, are often the cause of later disturbances of potency. And urination, is for some individuals an emotional equivalent for ejaculation. Such facts make more plausible the psycho-analytic discovery that, even in normal individuals, part of the sexual impulse is derived from urethral sources and part of the urethral impulse from sexual sources.

2224. *Pregenital and genital impulses.*

Although in the last sections we have seen that the barriers between oral, anal, urethral, and genital impulses are not so definite as used to be supposed, we must not forget that they all originally satisfied distinct needs. A rhythmical contraction of the stomach

[1] Havelock Ellis, *Studies in the Psychology of Sex*, iii, 60 ff.
[2] Ferenczi, *Versuch einer Genitaltheorie.*

F

walls, a weight on the bowels, a pressure on the bladder, and the presence of sexual substances, produce different stimuli and different needs. But Nature, with a greater regard for economy than for Victorian aesthetics, has as far as possible adapted reactions to each in the service of the others. Thus the child may be erotically excited by pregenital interests, and the adult may revert to them either as fixed perversions or as exciting preliminaries to the normal act of coitus.

225. *The aggressive impulse.*

The acquisitive tendency of the term sexual was not even exhausted by its supposed inclusion of oral, anal and urethral impulses. At one time it also threatened to absorb hate as a form of sadism. Possibly owing to a reaction against this monistic tendency, Freud, in his later works, has developed a dualistic metapsychology in which there is eternal strife between the impulses of Eros and of Death. But under the term ' death impulse ' Freud seems to understand three different things which have little in common except their name. First, there is the general tendency of all living matter to decay and die ; secondly there is its tendency to react as long as, and only as long as it is stimulated and therefore to " seek " absence of stimulus; and, lastly, there is an aggressive impulse, which is sometimes inverted against the self. It is this aggressive impulse with which we are here concerned.

The psychic correlate of aggression is hate. This emotion does not appear to be a primary emotion comparable to that of love. For, while the love impulse

is ultimately due to the accumulation of sexual substances which can be relieved by a certain series of
reactions, it is difficult to imagine that there is any
similar periodic need which can only be relieved by
an act of hate.[1] It seems, therefore, more reasonable
to regard hate, like fear, as a reaction to a threat or
frustration rather than as an independent impulse
comparable to that of love.

Since the sexual impulse is the one which is the most
often frustrated, hate and aggressiveness most often
occur in its support. We may even find some grounds
for the view that after all hate is a derivative of sex.

2251. *Aggressive rivalry.*

Probably aggressiveness did not have many origins,
but was evolved for one purpose and afterwards utilized
for others. It must have come into the world as the
result of over-population, and it is still largely maintained by this cause, but it has become instinctive,
and would probably survive even if there were plenty
of everything to go round. There are three possible
origins of aggressiveness and hate—hunger, self-defence,
and sexuality. Aggressiveness is most conspicuous
among carnivora, and at first sight one might in consequence attribute to it an oral origin. But whereas
the males of almost all species (herbivora and carnivora)

---

[1] While the chemical substances which produce the sensual
need always stimulate when they have been accumulated in
sufficient quantity, the adrenalin and other substances, whatever
they are, which excite aggressiveness appear to be only ejected
into the blood stream when they are wanted, *i.e.* when there is
frustration.

are aggressive in their rutting season, only some (carnivora and the larger herbivora) are aggressive in self-defence, and a still smaller proportion (the carnivora) are also aggressive in pursuit of food. Hence it would seem that aggressive rivalry in rut is more general and more primitive than aggression in hunger or in danger.

2252. *Sexual aggression.*

The males of most species are aggressive to their mates as well as to their rivals, and it may be argued plausibly that aggressiveness of all forms was originally a derivative of the sexual impulse.

Biologists have suggested that the weapons which the males of so many species possess were first evolved to master the resistance of the females, and that they were only afterwards adapted for sexual combat and for self-protection.[1] The posture which a male bird adopts to excite its mate is the same as that which it employs to terrify its rival. And Elliot Howard has suggested that the posture and the corresponding impulse may have been evolved ' firstly as a means of arousing the requisite amount of pairing hunger in the female, secondly as a warning to intruders, and thirdly as a protection for the helpless offspring.'[2]

If, therefore, aggressiveness of all types is really an adaptation of a sexual impulse, we can easily understand why aggressive acts in dreams so often symbolize sexual acts. This kind of symbolization often

---

[1] Roheim, *Animism, Magic and the Divine King*, 1930, p. 250, from Hesse-Doflein, *Tierbau und Tierleben*, 1924.
Elliot Howard, *British Warblers*, ii, summary 8.

appears to be quite conscious among primitive people
Thus, for instance, among the Kiwai, 'on leaving
for war a man is sometimes given a medicine by his wife
consisting of a piece of ginger which she has kept for
some time in her vulva. In the fight he will chew a
little of it, spit the juice onto himself, saying : " My
wife, like lightning straight where vulva I go," that is
he attacks, he goes for the vulva like lightning.' [1]
Nothing could show more clearly than this quotation
that the savage, like the dreamer, treats an aggressive
attack on an enemy as equivalent to an aggressive sexual
assault. The implication that the one impulse is a
derivative of the other, which has been taken over
and adapted for another purpose, is very strong.

2253. *The impulse to castrate.*

It seems probable that the impulse to castrate the
rival is an instinctive part of the aggressive rivalry
of man. Psycho-analysts have discovered in the
unconscious of their patients a universal fear of castration, and a desire to castrate others. Probably the
desire is primary and the fear is mainly the fear of the
projected desire. It would undoubtedly facilitate the
acceptance of these discoveries by those who have not
made them if it could be shown that animals akin
to us have similar desires and fears. I have been told
by a French sportsman that dogs hunting stags often
attack their genital organs and that the stags stand
at bay to protect especially these parts. Also
that rabbits castrate hares when they interfere with

[1] Roheim, *op. cit.*, p. 20.

the does. These observations have been contradicted by other naturalists whom I have questioned, so that I do not know whether they are genuine or mere current superstition. We usually only attribute falsely to others desires which we ourselves possess, whether we are conscious of them or disown them. If therefore the belief that animals castrate each other is only a superstition, it is still evidence that the desires exist in the men who believe them so readily. But if the observations are correct, they would prove what psycho-analysts should expect—namely that the desire to castrate or injure the genitals of a rival is an innate impulse not confined to man.

Apart from psycho-analytical evidence it is not hard to collect some independent confirmation of the existence of such an impulse in man. There are stories of medieval knights who, when they were prostrate beneath their enemy and about to receive the *coup de grace*, saved themselves by inflicting a mortal wound on the genitals of their opponents. Boxers in a state of panic have been known to defend themselves in a similar manner, in spite of the strong taboo against hitting below the belt. And I remember seeing small boys at school spontaneously discover this method of defence or attack.

If we may suppose that such an innate impulse does exist it may have been evolved by adapting a pre-existing homosexual sadism for the purpose. Among women the tendency to suck the male organ is so common that it should probably be regarded less as a perversion than as an instinct, which, like that of related animals, has been evolved to excite the male. Often this tendency among women is fused with sadism to form the desire to bite off the penis—an impulse which psycho-analysts find to be common in the unconscious, which is occasionally put in practice by the insane and even by the sane during the excitement of an orgasm, and which is hinted at in the myths and customs of primitive and ancient peoples.[1] Owing to cross inheritance it is quite likely that the males of many species have inherited this useless female impulse and have adapted it to the racially useful purpose of aggressive rivalry. This, at least, is to me the most plausible explanation of the desire to castrate rivals which is so conspicuous a feature in the unconscious of the males of our own species.

2254. *Carnivorous aggression.*

We have argued that the aggressiveness of the carnivore in pursuit of food is not likely to be primary, and that it is probably derived from sexual aggressiveness either directly or *via* the impulse of aggressive rivalry.

The hate of the carnivore is, however, especially

---

[1] In a discussion of the Psycho-Analytical Society one of the members stated that an insane patient had tried to bite his genitals, and that when she was frustrated in this attempt she had bitten him severely on the ankle. In a certain murder trial it transpired that the prisoner had killed his mistress in a fit of rage and pain after she had severely bitten his penis. And there are fertility rites like those in which the pregnant woman ' has to bite off the stalk of the ethrog (*Liebesapfel*) to facilitate parturition.' Roheim, *op. cit.*, 339.

interesting, because it throws light on the peculiar hatreds of men. The young kitten growls in an unearthly way over the first mouse or rat it catches. One feels, as one hears it, that the kitten has just discovered a new emotion, but an emotion which is instinctive, and is almost terrifying because it awakens a dim echo in one's own unconscious. I have read somewhere of a young tiger who, on being given meat for the first time, ' crunched it as if he hated it.' I can think of no better description of the emotion I mean. Hate in self-defence, in the defence of young, or in sexual rivalry, seems in comparison honest and not terrifying. But the hate of the kitten or of the young tiger, if it is fully realized, makes a most sinister impression ; for one feels instinctively that it is sadistic and that the young tiger hates the thing it loves. Other hates destroy threats of injuries or threats to means, but the canivore's hate destroys the means it seeks. We have seen that the gap between oral and genital love is less wide than used to be supposed. In the carnivore the object of oral love and of hate are the same. And this is but a step to the sadism in which the object of genital love and of hate are one.

Thus, although sexual aggressiveness is probably more ancient than the nutritional aggressiveness of the carnivore, there is little doubt that the developed sadism of the human race has borrowed much from oral sources. We shall see later that the ontogenesis of sadism in man occurs when the child is thwarted at his mother's breast. He then learns for the first time to hate the object he loves. Ever afterwards his loves may be sullied with hate and his hates with love. For the oral hate may contribute to genital love and the oral love to aggressive rivalry. All sadists have fantasies which approach to cannibalism; the Maenads of the Dionysiac revels found raw human flesh a deliciously licentious diet, and one occasionally hears of Hungarian gipsies[1] or of a Hanoverian butcher[2] who have made the same discovery.

226. *The self-preservative impulse.*

The concept of the sexual impulse has been still further widened by the argument that even the instinct of self-preservation, which was always supposed to be distinct from the instinct of reproduction, is really a derivative of self-love, or narcissism, which is itself a sexual derivative. In order to find out how far this view is justified we must try to define narcissism and follow its development.

Narcissism is obviously akin to positive self-feeling, and this affect seems to have been originally identical with a sense of sexual potency. It is an emotion which is typical of the stag or the stallion in the rutting season, or of the peacock which is endeavouring to excite the hen. It must therefore be much the same feeling as the sexual appetite of the male. This appetite we have defined as made up of the sensation of a need plus a sensation of the preliminary means plus an anticipation of the final means.[3] There is a confidence in appetite which is not present in desire. For, in

---

[1] In Kaschau, 1929.   [2] The Harmann case.
[3] *Cf.* Chap. ii, 2.

desire, the mate is not secured but only anticipated, whereas, in appetite, only the bodily erotic sensations, or final means, remain unrealized, though they are vividly anticipated. It is just this confidence of appetite which seems the chief constituent of that positive self-feeling which is so quickly shattered by an unlooked-for rebuff. William James in his account of shame, speaks of " that something in me . . . which a moment ago I felt inside of me, big and strong and lusty, but now weak, contracted and collapsed."[1] Surely these expressions reveal with unexampled clearness the sexual origin of positive self-feeling.

Although, in most species, this sort of arrogance seems to be confined to the male sex, in the human race women often notoriously display it more than men. The reason for this appears to be that the females of our species inherit or acquire an unusually large share of male impulses, which, whether retained or projected, are inverted towards their own persons. The normal woman disowns her masculine impulses and projects them upon her partner, so that, although she is herself their object and cannot be rebuffed by them, she is still dependent upon her capacity to excite another person to reflect her own desires. But there are other women who do not disown their masculine affection for themselves, so that they are independent of others. It is this positive self-feeling, which comes of choosing the self as the loved object, that is called narcissism.

Among men, those who are most narcissistic are those who have a strong component of feminine homosexual-

[1] James, *Principles of Psychology*, i, 321-2.

ity, and who have, in consequence, become one of the most satisfying objects of their own inverted desires. The less they have projected their impulses, the more narcissistically autonomous they are.

Narcissism is thus present when the self is selected as a sexual means. We have next to discover what connection it has with self-preservation. We may say at once that self-preservation in its simplest form, the innate or acquired impulse to avoid injuries, must have had an independent origin. But narcissism may well have been adapted by evolution to assist another impulse, and it is not difficult to see how this has come about. Self-preservation was originally determined by fear of injury to the self ; but, if the self is also the loved object, a threat of destruction to the self is also a threat of the loss of the loved object. And this perhaps explains that haunting fear of death or mutilation which has been so great an aid to self-preservation. Narcissism, however, does not contribute to the avoidance of all injuries, but only to the avoidance of those that involve death or mutilation. The narcissist is often also masochistic, where the pain does not involve a permanent loss. Self-preservation is thus a fusion of a non-sexual with a sexual impulse. It is a combination of the fear of injury with the fear of the loss of a sexual means.

227. *Love.*

In a former section we have discussed some of the contributions to the sexual impulse. But love includes something more than a simple impulse of generation reinforced by direct pre-genital desires. This extra factor which has so far eluded us is a sense of unity with the loved subject. In a later section we shall argue that this sense of unity between lovers depends upon a bisexual disposition which makes possible the projection and introjection of impulses from one partner to the other.[1] But here we may mention the role which narcissism appears to play in this process

Narcissism is in the main responsible for self-consciousness, for interest not only in one's own body but in one's own thoughts. Since man lost his anœstrum he is always in a state of subliminal or open sexual need, and, since his fellows restrict his otherwise limitless promiscuity, he has to fall back to a great extent upon self-love. This makes him body-conscious and introspective, and so he comes to learn about himself and to be the only kind of animal which is also a psychologist.

We are thus all narcissistic when we are not in love, but when we are in love we lose our narcissism and love someone else instead. The narcissist loves himself and enjoys in his own person both a masculine and a feminine role, and a narcissistic phase undoubtedly contributes much to bring out the latent sexuality belonging to the other sex, which everyone inherits. The narcissistic male enjoys both loving himself and being loved by himself.[2] When he afterwards falls in love with an independent object, this new person

---

[1] *Cf.* Chap. v, 3.

[2] *e.g.* He may first fall in love with his own limbs and movements as he postures naked before a glass and then suddenly become aware of the feminine thrill of being loved.

is required not only as an object of the previously inverted masculine impulses, but also as an object in whose person the feminine impulses which have been brought out in the narcissistic phase can be enjoyed by proxy. This is why the ex-narcissist cannot fully enjoy the excitement of love unless he feels that his partner also enjoys her role. For the feminine role is almost as important to him as the masculine one, but he can no longer enjoy it in his own person and can only satisfy it by empathy.

Freud distinguishes between an object love, which has been in this way derived from a narcissistic love, and an object love which does not have this derivation. But I think these differences are only differences of degree. A love unpreceded by any narcissism, and in which the loved object was in no sense a substitute for the self, would, I think, be defective in sympathy with, or understanding of, its object. For we must learn by our own narcissism to take an interest in and understand our own psychology before we can hope to take an interest in and understand the psychology of others. And for this reason women and men who have passed through a strong narcissistic or homo-sexual phase, are more sympathetic and understanding than other people.

The strong protective impulse which women display towards their young is also largely derived from a transference of a narcissistic self-love to their offspring. Such impulses are not confined to the females of our species. If I am right, narcissism, which was originally a by-product of an accidental bisexuality, has been adapted by evolution not only to contribute a large factor to self-preservation but also to normal love and to the preservation of the young.

It would seem probable that the cross inheritance of impulses belonging to the other sex which forms such an important part of the love of man is also utilized in the courting habits of animals. The males of apes and monkeys may often be observed to present their posteriors to the females when courting them.[1] The female is, perhaps, thereby incited to imitate this gesture, and so to give the male his opportunity. Small boys who have not yet learnt modesty sometimes adopt an identical procedure to induce a small girl to expose herself. Now the presentation of the posterior is a female instinct in monkeys. But they are excited to it more readily when the males give them an example. Thus the male monkey's courting gesture of presenting his posterior would seem to be a female impulse which he has inherited and which has been fixed and adapted as a means of exciting the female. Certain monkeys have evolved bright colouring on their buttocks to increase the effectiveness of the gestures. Possibly the exhibitionism of the peacock and of the males of many birds may also be due to the adaptation to the purpose of male courting of a similar female posture.

'Among moor-hens and great crested grebes sometimes what Selous terms " functional hermaphroditism " occurs and the females play the part of the male to-

[1] Darwin draws a parallel between such behaviour and the courting postures of peacocks. *Descent of Man*, supplementary note on Sexual Selection in relation to Monkeys.

wards their male companions, and then repeat the sexual act with a reversion to the normal order, the whole to the satisfaction of both parties.'[1] The cross-inherited male impulses of the females seem here to be clearly adapted to the excitement of the males. Such facts suggest that the sense of unity between lovers is not confined to the human species, and that pairs of apes and birds, at least, may not only mutually reflect each other's sexual excitement but that they may also sympathetically enjoy it.

23. The primal family.

We may conclude this attempt to describe some of our instincts and to sketch a reconstruction of their development, by a speculative picture of the psychology of our ancestors at a time when they had but slightly diverged from their cousins the ancestors of the anthropoid apes.

There is some difference of opinion as to whether primal man (Urmensch) lived in families containing one adult male or in herds containing several. I will sketch my own version of the psycho-analytic view, but it should be understood that it is only a speculation.

231. Herds.

The larger carnivores, like lions and tigers, whose food supply is scattered, who do not require assistance in killing game, and who are not preyed upon by still larger carnivores, are usually solitary. But herbivores,

[1] E. Selous, The Zoologist, 1902, p. 196, quoted by Havelock Ellis, Studies in the Psychology of Sex, iii, 233.

like deer or horses, whose food supply is plentiful and who require protection, and carnivores like wolves, who require assistance in killing game, are usually gregarious. The Eo-anthropoids, or pre-men, were largely herbivores, who were preyed upon by other animals, and who in so far as they were carnivores, probably required assistance in running down their prey. Thus it was in their interest to be gregarious, and we may suppose that they, at least once, lived in a gregarious condition.

232. *Families.*

Food supply and self-defence are not the only conditions that determine the size of an animal group. Sexual jealousy is a dividing factor more powerful even than shortage of food. A herd of deer, for example, during the rutting season splits into a polygamous family and a band of young males who hover round and try to defeat the leader or to steal his wives. Therefore, since the rutting season splits the herd into a family, we might expect that those species who have lost their anoestrum and live in a condition of perpetual rut would also lose all gregarious stability. The evidence of naturalists does not altogether support this view, for many of the apes and monkeys, who have lost their anoestrum, still live in herds. But the gorilla, which is most akin to man, does seem to display the family organization which psycho-analysts would expect.[1]

If, however, we study the exceptions more closely, they seem after all to prove the rule. In a collection

[1] For a summary of psycho-analytical contributions to animal psychology see Storfer, *Psychoanalytische Bewegung*, iii, *Uber psychoanalytische Tierpsychologie.*

of monkeys of both sexes it appears that the right of intercourse is confined to one male, and that the rest are homosexual. If an enterprising youngster presumes to attack the leader and is defeated, he immediately presents his posterior like a female, and is ridden by his victor.[1] We may therefore understand why these young males can live on in the same family. They are tolerated and perhaps even loved by the leader because they do not threaten his monopoly. And they have a homosexual consolation for their restraint.

Freud has argued that the clan basis of human society depends for its existence on unconscious homosexuality. Whether the ancestors of man passed directly from the herd organization to that of the clan, or whether they passed through an intermediate family organization, cannot yet be determined with certainty. But they were more comparable in fierceness and courage to the gorilla than to the social monkeys, and it seems probable that, like the gorilla, they were once too jealous to tolerate each other in a herd.[2]

2321. *The loss of the anoestrum.*

We have seen that the loss of the anoestrum was probably the cause of the break up of the old herd organization, and for its displacement either by the polygamous family or by a pseudo-herd in which

[1] Zuckerman, *The Social Behaviour of Apes and Monkeys*, paper read to the British Psycho-Analytical Society, February, 1930 (now published in this Library).

[2] Recent observations have suggested that the gorilla may be a social animal after all. If so, is his social organization communal or aristocratic? The conflicting evidence perhaps might be explained if we suppose that he is in the transitional phase between the patriarchal family and the aristocratic clan.

G

all but the dominant male were homosexual. We may briefly consider the possible causes of this loss of an inter-rutting period which has been so important in our evolution. Probably it was due to the adoption of the upright position and the development of the sense of sight at the expense of that of smell. In those animals in which the sense of smell is highly developed, the most important erotic stimulus is olfactory. Even where there is no natural periodicity in the sexual need of the male, the sexual appetite tends to lie dormant until it is excited by the presence of the preliminary means. Where this preliminary means is the sight of the female the stimulus is always present, but where it is a smell which she only periodically emits, the male is only periodically excited, or at least the excitement in the intervening periods is greatly lessened. We may conclude therefore that the loss of the anoestrum, or inter-rutting period, originated in the loss of the importance of the sense of smell.[1]

2322. *Parricide.*

Even before the loss of the anoestrum, there must have been great fratricidal fights within the herd during the rutting season, but after the anoestrum had dwindled away, these fights probably became unceasing until the herd organization became impossible and its place was taken by the family.

Civil war was not, however, terminated by the family organization, but merely rendered less common. In the herd it was permanent and fratricidal; in the family occasional and parricidal. The young males

[1] Freud, *Das Unbehagen in der Kultur*, 62 f.

must have lived with the family for security until they were sexually mature. But when they reached the age of puberty they would be likely to be driven out to live in male bands, or perhaps to acquire wives by stealth. In every such family, however, there must have come a time when the leader grew old, or was injured, or lost his strength. Perhaps the first sign of the coming tragedy was a decline in sexual potency. The numerous women were no longer satisfied and would be inclined to look wistfully at the young males who now, more than ever, hovered round the camp. Friction and fights must have become more common until at last they broke in and killed their father. Dim records of these revolutions are to be found in the mythology of almost every people. Osiris of the Egyptians, and Ombure the Giant Crocodile God of the Fan, have been interpreted by Roheim as personifications of innumerable primal fathers who had been slain by their sons.[1] Among the Shilluk, the king was killed when he could no longer satisfy his harem.[2] This, too, seems like the survival in ritual of a parricidal habit.

We may suppose that, even at the time of these parricidal wars, the periodicity of a rutting season and an anoestrum had not completely died out. The males were no longer dependent upon the erotic stimulus of smell, but their sexual appetite was doubtless increased when the female was in that condition, which perhaps corresponded to what is now the menstrual period.

---

[1] Roheim, *Nach dem Tode des Urvaters*, Imago, ix, and *Australian Totemism*.

[2] Frazer, *Golden Bough*, ed. 3, iv, 17-26.

The later taboo on menstruation suggests that the attraction of this condition is still present in the unconscious.[1] The final break-up of each family must therefore have occurred during one of those periods of erotic maxima which corresponded to the former rutting season.[2] Even at the present time statistics show that the maxima for conceptions and for parricides occur together, in May-June and in October.[3]

2323. Incest.

There is one other factor of first importance for the subsequent history of man which contributed to the extreme animus of these early battles. The infancy period of the human child is relatively long, and in a state of nature it is suckled by its mother for several years. We have seen that infantile oral impulses form a large part of the later sexual impulse. Thus it comes about that an object relation developed at the oral phase forms the basis of subsequent affections, and the human boy acquires that incestuous fixation which is so regular a feature of his unconscious. At the time of the primal family this preference for the mother as the mate was probably conscious. If so, the exiled brothers would tend to attack their own father in preference to the leader of some other group.

2324. Cannibalism.

There is a good deal of indirect psycho-analytical and

---

[1] Daly, *Der Menstruationskomplex*, Imago, xiv.
[2] Roheim, *Australian Totemism.*
[3] Havelock Ellis, *Studies in the Psychology of Sex*, ed. 3, i, 150.

anthropological evidence to lead us to believe that the primal father was eaten as well as slain. Thus, for example, the totem animal of primitive people is often not only revered and protected as a father, but killed and eaten as a sacrament.

It seems just possible that Eoanthropus was at first almost purely herbivorous, and that he learnt his carnivorous habits at home. The primitive taboos of meats in the couvade have been interpreted by Reik as taboos of filiophagy,[1] and Roheim has argued that those during the mourning period were originally taboos of patrophagy.[2] Many herbivorous animals make one exception to their usual diet and occasionally eat their young. Pigs and rabbits are notorious in this respect, and monkeys will at least eat those of their young who die. Such accidents are probably due to an inadequate extension of the instinct of most female mammals to eat their placenta and to lick their young. Possibly the males through cross inheritance might have developed this disposition and so paved the way for a filiophagous perversion. If so, the primal father, like Chronos, may sometimes have eaten his children. But those who escaped doubtless lived to express their gratitude like Zeus, who castrated his father, or like Ngurangurane, who ate him.

[1] Reik, *Probleme der Religionspsychologie.*
[2] Roheim, *Australian Totemism.*

CHAPTER IV

THE DEVELOPMENT OF CULTURAL IMPULSES

IT seems to me probable that the innate impulses of the civilized individual of to-day are not materially different from those of primal man, and that our gentler nature is due less to evolution than to the slow accumulation of a culture which is not inherited but which we acquire partly through the threats of our elders and partly by imitating them. We differ from these remote ancestors not so much in any positive impulses, but in the possession of a colossal system of inhibitions. Unlike many psychologists of the psycho-analytic school, I think that these are hardly, if at all, innate, but the product of our social environment. Thus I believe that if a colony of infants could be transported to an uninhabited island, and by some miracle grow up untended, they would soon break up into small families each dominated by one male ; that the sons of the next generation, impelled by innate incestuous impulses, would endeavour to castrate, kill, and eat their fathers ; and that, if they were successful, they would fight among themselves until the herd again split into families, each led by one young male who would live for a space in the fulfilment of his incestuous ambition.

Such, at least, was probably the behaviour of the species from which we are descended, whose instincts may still be detected in our own unconsciousnesses. The origin and maintenance of the inhibitions which repress these impulses are undoubtedly dependent upon an innate bisexual disposition which we share with apes and monkeys. But the inhibitions themselves I ascribe to culture rather than to instinct.

The primary function of culture is thus to build up and to transmit inhibitions ; but it also fulfils a secondary function in developing and transmitting suitable sublimations for the distorted expression of what it has repressed. We may therefore divide our discussion of the development of cultural impulses into two parts which we may label cultural inhibitions and cultural sublimations.

I. *Cultural inhibitions.*

II. *From family to clan.*

The ancestors of man, we have argued, lived first in herds and then in families. But the family itself gave place to the clan. In the last chapter we outlined a possible development of the herd into the family. In the present section we have to try to reconstruct the development of the family into the clan. But while the evolution of the herd into the family was perhaps mainly due to the evolution of an innate character, namely the loss of the anoestrum, I believe that the development of the family into the clan was made possible by the acquisition of inhibitions which are transmitted by tradition.

I can submit no direct evidence for the theory I am about to expound, but nevertheless I think it is a legitimate deduction from the psychology of primal man. This psychology we still have in our unconscious, and by deducting the acquisitions of culture, we can expose it fairly accurately. It is of a type which is compatible with the family organization outlined in the last chapter, but quite incompatible with the organization of the herd. We have seen reason to believe that at a still earlier stage the ancestors of man lived in herds.[1] But those who, like Trotter, believe that we have passed straight from the herd to the clan organization, without passing through the stage of the Primal family, not only neglect the incestuous and parricidal tendencies which, after the loss of the anoestrum, must have made the herd organization unstable, but also fail to notice that the clan is more similar to the family than to the herd in everything except numbers.

We start, then, with the assumption that man once lived in families, and that the family is still his natural unit, the unit into which he would inevitably relapse if it were not for the maintenance of cultural inhibitions. We have now to ask how the clan organization developed and how it is maintained. In answering this question, psychology is almost our only guide.

12. *The transference of sexual and aggressive impulses.*

It appears to be a general, though regrettable, attribute of man that he cannot combine into groups except

[1] *Cf.* Chap. iii, 231.

in hostility to other groups. Co-operation is thus a consequence of, rather than an alternative to, competition. The brothers of the Primal family co-operated to slay their father ; but they competed with each other after he was dead. The parties of the French revolution combined to destroy the aristocrats, but slaughtered each other as soon as they were successful. The Mensheviks and Bolsheviks similarly behaved towards each other. But conflicting factions can be united in the face of a common foe. For this reason, statesmen, whether they aim at protecting an old government or consolidating a new one, sometimes invent imaginary dangers and offences to divert the aggressiveness of the people from themselves. In this way they provide an outlet for that aggressiveness, which was primarily evolved to be of use in sexual combats, which is now the hidden fire below the mountain of civilization, and which from time to time destroys it.

The sexual inhibitions of civilization have diverted the longings and rivalries of sexuality into the economic sphere. Many of the luxuries which men seek, or envy each other for possessing, can be shown to be substitutes for more direct sexual means. Thus economic discontent is the modern form of the rivalry of the brothers of the Primal family. Aggressive imperialism as a cure for internal discontent is now less openly advocated by statesmen ; it has many obvious disadvantages and it is at least limited by the number of nations there are left to conquer ; but it is still the most effective prophylactic which has been invented. In our own country it has been resuscitated under the disguised form of Empire Free Trade as an alternative to socialist taxation. Even the communist rulers of revolutionary France, in the past, and of Russia, in the present, have had to adopt their revolutionary crusades to divert the aggressiveness of the people from themselves. Probably a similar, though less conscious, policy converted Primal families into clans.

Perhaps an Ice Age drove great numbers of people into a country too small to support them.[1] But in any case an altered relation between population and food supply must have caused family to fight with family for the possession of a hunting territory, and diverted internal strife to a foreign foe. Two transferences of impulse which are interdependent may nevertheless be distinguished ; the transference of the possessive impulse from its original sexual object to the hunting territory, and the transference of the aggressive impulse from the sexual rival to the family of strangers who threatened this territory.

Among many animals the sense of property is strongly developed. Wolves and baboons fight for hunting or feeding grounds,[2] and certain male birds will fight for a nesting territory before the arrival of the females provides a direct sexual incentive to these battles. Elliot Howard[3] has suggested that the aggressive

[1] Freud and Ferenczi have suggested that the Ice Age had something to do with repression.
[2] Carveth Read, *Origin of Man*, 44, 56-9.
[3] *British Warblers*, ii, summary 8.

postures of birds may first have been evolved 'as a means of arousing the requisite amount of pairing hunger in the female,' and have been later adapted as a warning to intruders who threaten the mate, or the nesting territory before the arrival of the mate, and as a defence for the young. If he is right, aggressiveness in general is perhaps not only a development of the aggressiveness of sexual rivalry, but the aggressiveness of sexual rivalry is itself ultimately a modification of an aggressive preliminary to the sexual act directed not to a rival but to the mate herself.[1] But at the moment we are only interested in the progress from defence of the mate to defence of the nesting territory, that is, in the extension of rivalry from the sexual to the economic sphere. If this extension has taken place in birds and other animals it is likely to have taken place in man also, though in man it may be a cultural rather than a racial development. Psycho-analysis has shown that earth or land is a common dream-symbol of a woman, more especially the mother, and whether this symbolism is innate or acquired, its existence proves the ease with which a possessive impulse can be transferred from a mother to a strip of land. Princes have often rebelled against their fathers in order to usurp their place, and such events are a common theme of romance. Rank has shown that in such real or fantasied revolts the conscious motive is often a transparent substitute for the more fundamental unconscious sexual rivalry.[2] Among the sons of the Primal family a similar transference of the

[1] See Chap. iii, 2251.   [2] *Das Inzest-Motiv.*

possessive impulse from their mother to their hunting territory must have arisen under the pressure of population upon the food supply.

This partial diversion of the sexual aim must have inevitably involved a partial diversion of the aggressiveness from the sexual rival to the common foe. Just as the threatened hunting ground became a symbol of the mother, so the invaders, or defenders, of the disputed land became symbols of the once hated father.[1] Father and sons thus came to tolerate each other as valuable allies ; the sons were less ready to attack their father, and the father was less ready to drive out his sons as soon as they were full grown.

13. *Puberty rites.*

We have argued that competition with other groups for hunting territories may have first enabled the sons of a primal family to transfer their aggressiveness from their own father to the leaders of these other groups. But such transferences of affects were unlikely to have alone secured the permanent stability of the clan, and in the intervals of external war the old internal strife must often have broken out. Fathers must have had many occasions to fear and hate their sons. Provoked by attempts at seduction, and following what we have seen some reason to believe may be a natural instinct, they may often have castrated them. Castration is the

---

[1] The transference of sexual desire from the mother to the women of the hostile family, which must also have taken place, would appear to be secondary to the transference of hate from the father to the leader of the other group.

earliest operation performed by man ; he performed it upon animals as soon as he began to domesticate them, and before he performed it upon animals he may have performed it upon his sons. First occasionally, and then as a tribal custom, the older generation very likely emasculated a certain proportion of the youths. The puberty rites of primitive people to-day all suggest such earlier customs. In one tribe, a testicle is cut out ;[1] in others the youths are subincised or circumcised, and in yet others, a tooth is knocked out or some other mutilation performed which, psycho-analysts tell us, symbolizes castration.[2]

One purpose of the puberty rite is thus to terrorize the younger generation, for it symbolizes castration and forcibly suggests the real punishment which will follow any interference with forbidden women. This purpose is no longer conscious, but it is still admitted that such rites teach the boys a healthy respect for the tribal taboos. The real castration remains, however, among many people the penalty for interference with the wives of older or more important men. Thus, ' In Egypt castration was the penalty for adultery, while in India a Sudra who committed adultery with the wife of an Arya, or who insolently made water on a high-caste man, suffered amputation of the penis ; and a Brahman who dishonoured the bed of his teacher had, as one of the three modes of death offered him, the option of himself amputating his penis and scrotum, and of then advancing

[1] Frazer, *Belief in Immortality*, iii, 146.
[2] For further examples of such rites see Otto Stoll, *Geschlechtsleben in der Völkerpsychologie*.

holding them in his hand, to the south-west (the direction of Nirrti, " Destruction ") until he should fall dead.'[1] There can be little doubt that the puberty rites include representations of such penalties.

Thus three causes contribute to permit families to grow into clans—the partial transference of sexual impulses from sisters and mother to a threatened hunting territory,[2] the partial transference of hate from the father to rival hunters, and the intimidation in puberty rites of the young generation by the old. These causes may have been sufficient to *suppress* the incestuous and parricidal impulses which threatened to destroy the clan, but I do not think that alone they would have been sufficient to *repress* them. Impulses which are already partially diverted may be suppressed by fear of retaliation, but I think that they would remain conscious, and that something more than this sort of fear is required to convert suppression into repression, and to prevent, not only the execution of a desire, but also its discovery by the self.

14. *Homosexuality.*

It is well known that apes and monkeys are bisexual and that the males frequently mount or present themselves to other males. Such perversions appear to be most common in those individuals who have not secured mates. But the feminine homosexual response of presentation is commonly evoked by any aggressive

---

[1] Gray, *Encyclopaedia of Religion and Ethics.*
[2] And to the women of other groups.

attack.[1] We may thus conclude that, in monkeys and primates, homosexuality is both a relief for normal deprivation and an alternative to self-defence. Exactly parallel, though less explicit, behaviour can be observed in our own species. In the negative Œdipus complex, the son who feels himself thwarted by his father becomes inverted towards him and in this way seeks a consolation for what he has given up. It is this mechanism which is at the basis of religion and morality.[2] The disposition to it is innate, but its product is an acquired culture which is transmitted by tradition. We have now to reconstruct the beginning of these cultural inhibitions.

The younger generation of a primitive group were intimidated by their elders and lived in abstinence, deprived of the normal means of satisfying their sexual needs. We have seen that a sexual means is also a means to the removal of various other needs or threats, and that the permanent fixation to such an object is mainly due to these secondary functions which it fulfils.[3] The mother is needed originally because she fulfils real wants, and later because she is a protector against all sorts of imaginary injuries and needs. And, mainly because she is needed for these secondary purposes she is also selected as the primary sexual object when the sexual need develops and coordinates so many other impulses which once had independent uses. When the family was threatened by other families, the father became protector as well as rival. He thus became a means to many needs which the mother used to satisfy

---

[1] Cf. Chap. iii, 232.   [2] Cf. Chap. vi, 21, 22.
[3] Chap. iii, 22.

alone. The father who deprived the sons of the mother became at the same time an object which could largely take her place. Sons thus began to love their fathers and to repress their rivalry. There is no terror greater than the threat of the loss of a means, and after the father became the only permitted means, the child's dread of being left by his mother grew into the dread of losing his father.[1] And this fear was very real because the sons knew dimly that the fathers' chief danger was their own undying hate. Therefore they repressed this hate and tried to forget that it existed. Such at least is the origin of repression in the child of to-day ; we may suppose that the same mechanisms operated in the same way in primeval times.

If this argument is correct, the main motive for the repression of incestuous and parricidal impulses was not so much fear of the father as love of him. Ultimately both these motives may be reduced to fear ; but whereas fear of the father's retaliation is fear of a possible indirect consequence of attacking him, fear of losing him is fear of a direct consequence of too successful an attack.

15. *The transmission of inhibitions.*

The repression of parricidal and incestuous desires, once it is acquired, is transmitted as the most important part of culture, even if it has not become innate. Some of the conditions which first produced it are still operative

---

[1] Roheim has argued (*Nach dem Tode des Urvaters*, Imago, ix,) that the sacramental eating of a Father God owes its existence to the transference of oral impulses from the mother to the father.

and it has itself produced others which take the place of the rest. There are still diversions of rivalry which attract aggressiveness from its original object. Among primitive people there is still the possibility of inter-tribal war. And even among civilized nations a satisfactory alternative to imperialism as a diversion of revolutionary ardour has yet to be found. Competition in business or sport or even in science do something to satisfy our aggressiveness, but to those who have a limited capacity for sublimation they are poor substitutes for the real thing.

There are not only still non-sexual diversions of sexual rivalry, but there are also still threats to assist the suppression of that part of the original aggressiveness which has not been diverted. The father himself is no longer so brutal as he was, but real father-substitutes are found in the older generation, the aristocracy, public opinion, or in the chief or king, and imaginary father-substitutes in totems or gods, which are all feared and believed capable of avenging a transgression of the fundamental taboos.[1] These taboos were once taboos of incest and parricide, but they have been widened to forbid the extended incest of endogamy or the extended parricide of the murder of a kinsman. Lastly, each, normally educated individual develops a conscience or super-ego which is formed by the introjection of the parental imago. But the formation of the super-ego depends upon that transference of love from the mother to the father which helped to originate repression and is now the main factor which maintains it.

[1] *Cf.* Money-Kyrle, *The Meaning of Sacrifice*, Part 1, Chap. vi.

H

We saw that it was originally the father's threats operating against already weakened incestuous and parricidal tendencies which produced a state of deprivation favourable to the transference of inhibited love from the mother to the father. There are two factors which determine a child's love for another person—the extent to which alternative objects are inaccessible, and the extent to which the new object himself solicits this love. The child's need of love is so great that he will love anyone, however brutal, if there is no alternative, but, if there are alternatives, a candidate must make himself attractive before he can hope to win the child's affection. At the beginning of repression, the father's brutality probably secured the condition of complete deprivation necessary for the transference of affection to himself. But the son who has once learnt to love his father will be likely to transfer this feeling to his own son, who symbolizes his father. Such a father will be less jealous of his sons and will not deprive them so completely of their mother. But this deprivation will be less necessary, for he will attract rather than compel their affection. Some deprivation there will still be, but it will be largely exerted by the mother, who is herself under the influence of the incest taboo, and every snub which she inflicts will still further facilitate a transference of affection from herself to her husband. Many fathers are dimly aware of this and make the most of their opportunities.

16. *The super-ego.*
Love of the father, built up in this way, is a far stronger

represser of parricidal impulses than threats. But the threats reappear in a new and still more powerful form, for they no longer come directly from the father but from the super-ego in a manner which we must now try to understand. Repressed impulses may be either completely unconscious or they may be merely disowned and projected. When an impulse is projected, someone, other than the self is imagined as the agent of the desired act. The act is still anticipated as in a conscious desire, but it is thought of as performed by someone else. The child who has repressed his incestuous impulses no longer consciously imagines himself making an attack upon his mother ; but he may still imagine the attack being made by someone else. In fact, he imagines it so vividly that he may afterwards believe that he has actually witnessed such an attack, and, in the early stages of psycho-analysis, analysts were led astray by such pseudo-memories and were convinced that children must nearly always have opportunities of witnessing a parental coitus. In exactly the same way, the child's aggressive impulses may be projected. If he has transferred part of his love for his mother to his father, his father becomes almost as necessary to him as his mother, and the thought of losing him is unbearable. The aggressive impulses are therefore disowned and projected. Many little boys show an exaggerated fear lest some harm should happen to their fathers because they have projected their own hate and feel vaguely that their fathers are threatened in some mysterious way they know not how. Often this aggressiveness is projected upon the father himself, and the concept of a brutal father is developed, which the father himself has done nothing to earn—except in so far as his very tenderness has forced his son to disown his hate and to project it. At the same time as the aggressiveness is projected it may also be inverted and directed towards the self. Then the original aggressiveness is exactly reversed. The fantasy of the child hating, killing, and castrating his father is converted into the fantasy of being hated, killed, or castrated by him. Both fantasies are probably repressed, but they continue to exist in different layers of the unconscious.

The final event in the development of the super-ego is the separation of this concept of the father, which was originally formed by the projection of the son's own repressed desires, from the real person. Instead it becomes identified with a tribal deity, who is jealous of the tribal laws, or with a mere vague personification of these laws or of public opinion, or it may survive as the voice of conscience from which even the atheist cannot escape. It is responsible for those inhibitions which, till now, have alone rendered culture possible ; but it is also responsible for neuroses when it is too powerful to permit satisfactory alternatives for what it has repressed. Once it is formed it cannot be destroyed. It may be modified by psycho-analysis and rendered more humane, but I have never heard of an analyst who complained that the super-ego of a patient had weakened to a dangerous extent. But though the super-ego cannot be destroyed it is not, I think, an innate structure, and a loss in the continuity of culture might well allow it to remain unformed. The main problem of the psycho-analytical educationalist is to discover under what conditions it can be developed strongly enough to protect the older generation, yet not too strongly to cause neurosis.

2. *Cultural sublimations.*

After this brief consideration of the development and maintenance of cultural inhibitions we may turn to consider the development of cultural sublimations.

The three most conspicuous types of cultural sublimations are magic, art and science. These all owe their energy, though not their utility, to repressed impulses which they satisfy symbolically. A symbol, we have seen[1], is a false threa or an inadequate means, which irrelevantly or inadequately resembles what is unconsciously avoided or sought. Thus a symbolic action is really an irrelevant avoidance or an inadequate seeking. But in the psycho-analytic terminology only those irrelevant or inadequate acts are symbolic which are substitutes for something which is repressed and not merely undiscovered.

We may note in passing that not merely positive desires but also fears are repressed. Repressed fears, however, owe their existence to repressed desires. Thus an unconscious fear of castration is an inevitable complement of an unconscious incestuous desire. Such desires and fears may give rise respectively to positive and negative sublimations.[2]

Symbolic acts may be rationalized or not, and if they

[1] *Cf.* Chap. ii, 121, 3112.
[2] *Cf.* Chap. v, 42, 43 ; vii, 1.

are rationalized, they may be rationalized falsely or truly. To rationalize a symbolic act is to suppose that it satisfies some impulse other than that which really evoked it. If it does satisfy this other impulse, it is rationalized truly ; if not, it is rationalized falsely. If an impulse is rationalized falsely, it is irrelevant or inadequate twice over, once because it avoids or seeks something which inadequately or irrelevantly resembles something which is unconsciously sought or avoided, and once because it does not even fulfil its secondary conscious purpose. Magic is made up of symbolic acts which are falsely rationalized ; art, of symbolic acts which are not rationalized at all; and science, of symbolic acts which are truly rationalized.

In this section we shall say something about the development of magic, art, and science. They each comprise a collection of ready made sublimations, which the individual may imitate instead of inventing new sublimations of his own.

21. *Art.*

It has often been disputed whether art has developed from magic or magic from art. Both views are probably correct, but since art is not rationalized it is perhaps simpler than magic which is rationalized falsely.

The artist creates symbolically that which he has forbidden himself, but which he still unconsciously desires. If we cannot justify this formula in detail we can at least indicate some of the repressed feelings and desires (i.e. the latent content) which help to determine the artistic product (i.e. the manifest expression).

211. *Phallic and vaginal symbols.*

The late J. Warburton Brown, in an interesting paper,[1] has pointed out that the design of pictures and statues is very often either triangular or elliptical. Now the triangle and the ellipse in dreams and in mythology are well-known symbols of the phallus and the vagina, and Warburton Brown has inferred that these shapes have the same significance when they occur in the plastic arts. To anyone who is not a psycho-analyst this inference may seem to have the slenderest foundation, but Warburton Brown and Eckart von Sydow[2] have collected archaeological evidence that the statue has in fact historically evolved from the phallic column of early magic and religion, and the pictures which they reproduce of intermediate forms leave little doubt that the argument, is in the main, correct.

I think we may assume, therefore, that the pleasure which the artist or the spectator obtains from the creation or observation of a statue or a picture is often partly due to the phallic or vaginal symbolism of the design. Put crudely, this design may very well excite repressed desires either to exhibit one's own sexual organs or to observe those of others, and, although the desires themselves need not become conscious, the elation peculiar to them may escape the censor.

The feelings aroused by works of art are naturally more complicated than this, but there is no doubt that something of the kind forms a more important element

[1] ' Psycho-Analysis and Design in the Plastic Arts,' *International Journal of Psycho-Analysis*, x.
[2] *Primitive Kunst und Psychoanalyse.*

in the general emotion than is recognized. After all, we are evolved from pre-human ancestors, and it should not surprise us that the highest feelings of which we are capable are derived from those which are common also to animals. If the sexual impulse is innate it must be innately excited by shapes which resemble its objects, and the more it is repressed the less will it differentiate between relevant and irrelevant similarity, and the more will its peculiar emotions be divorced from the definite idea of these objects. In so far as it is still conscious, it is excited more by a personality than by a sex organ ; it may be excited in half conscious form as an emotion separated from a desire by the contemplation of shapes (*Gestalten*) resembling these organs which are hidden in the composition of a work of art.

Probably the plastic arts do not only awaken unconscious desires, but also satisfy them. Desires, however, which are satisfied by mere symbols cannot represent real needs. Therefore we must conclude that, in so far as works of art provide a genuine satisfaction, and not merely an excitation, they must evoke removals or avoidances of false threats. This function may be illustrated by the following example.

It is known that the burial-place of primitive religion is often a symbol of the womb, to which the dead king believed that he returned. There is a good deal of apparent evidence of the existence of a very fundamental desire in man to return to the place from which he was ejected at his birth, and Rank[1] and Ferenczi[2]

---

[1] *The Trauma of Birth.*   [2] *Versuch einer Genitaltheorie.*

have elaborated important theories about this supposed desire.[1] Psycho-analysts continually meet its apparent representation in dreams and fantasies, but at present they are undecided whether it is really a fundamental urge or whether it is itself the distorted representation of an incestuous coitus in which the whole body symbolizes the penis. But whether the fantasy of returning to the womb is a fundamental wish or whether it is merely a symbolic representation of the phantasy of incestuous coitus, the fact remains that it is extremely common. There is little doubt that, to the Egyptians and to many primitive peoples, the tomb was a symbol of the mother, and that the Pharaoh reconciled himself to his inevitable death with the belief that he was to return for ever to the place of bliss from whence he came, where all his needs would be satisfied and where he would be at peace for ever. When the old idea of the abode of the dead in the tomb began to give way to the idea of a celestial home, the vault of heaven acquired the same symbolic meaning. Thus in the Pyramid texts we read : ' King Teti is this eye of Re, that passes the night, is conceived and born every day. . . . His mother the sky bears him living every day like Re. He dawns with him in the east, he sets with him in the west, his mother Nut (the sky) is not void of him any day.'[3] The dead king is identified with Re and spends every night in the womb of his mother Nut, and even in the day she is not void of him. Thus not only the

---

[1] Cf. Chap. v, 21.   [2] Flügel, The Psycho-Analytic Study of the Family, Ch. viii.

[3] Breasted, Religion and Thought in Ancient Egypt, 1912, p. 123.

grave but also the celestial sphere is a symbol of the womb.[1]

There is no doubt that such beliefs were a real consolation to those who held them. But no real need can be satisfied by a mere symbol. Therefore the pleasure which we may attribute to the Egyptian king at the contemplation of his finished tomb was the pleasure of relief from neurotic anxiety.

Roheim has argued that the soul is often a phallic symbol and that death symbolizes castration. ' According to the Suk, a man's spirit at death passes into a snake. The Masai believe that the soul of a rich man or medicine-man turns into a snake as soon as the body rots. According to some tribes in Madagascar, at death a worm or lizard or serpent called *fanany* emerges from the putrefying body. The *fanany* contains the soul of the deceased.'[2] As Roheim points out, all these snakes, lizards, or worms are phallic symbols, ' but most convincing of all is the belief of the Romans in a genius. The genius is a serpent. Genius and Juno were in the same relation to each other as procreation and conception.'[3] In particular he argues that the Egyptian Ka was also a phallic symbol,[4] and it is certainly a curious coincidence that the fish which swallowed the

[1] In former times the king of the Shilluk, when no longer able to satisfy the sexual passions of his wives, was walled up in a hut with his head resting on the lap of a nubile virgin until both died of thirst and hunger (Frazer, *Golden Bough*, iv, 17-26). Possibly this rite satisfied, among other things, the fantasy of pre-natal regression.

[2] Roheim, *Animism, Magic, and the Divine King*, 1930, pp. 15-16.   [3] *Ib.* 17.   [4] *Ib.* 19.

phallus of Osiris was the same fish that transported the soul of the dead to the other world. If the soul is a phallic symbol, and the tomb or celestial sphere are symbols of the womb, the contemplation of the future relation of these objects must have helped to dispel the neurotic fear of death which symbolized castration. The Egyptian in this way avoided the fear of death and feared only that he would die unburied. Therefore the contemplation of his tomb or of his abode in the womb of his mother the Sky satisfied because it avoided a false threat. Warburton Brown has argued that 'designs in pictures and other forms of plastic art, represent primarily an attempt to call forth feelings which satisfy certain unconscious wishes connected with the idea of potency as a negation of the idea of castration.'[1] Possibly the artist sometimes derives the same consolation from the composition of a picture as the Pharaoh from the design of his tomb or from his concept of the sky.

From the tomb evolved the temple, and from the temple the house. But to point out a historical connection between two creations of man is not to prove that the later structure owes its existence to the same unconscious desires as its predecessor. There is, however, much psycho-analytical evidence that the house does in fact still symbolize the same thing that the tomb did to early man. An acquaintance of mine, for instance, who spends much of his leisure in designing imaginary houses, and who has analysed these fantasies, is convinced

[1] ' Psycho-Analysis and Design in the Plastic Arts,' *International Journal of Psycho-Analysis*, x, 28.

that they do satisfy the unconscious fantasy of prenatal regression. In some of the more extravagant designs of such buildings as underground Turkish baths, which were to form the background of singular erotic adventures, this meaning is very evident ; and from these fantasies there is a gradual transition to more practical schemes of restful interiors or secluded gardens. From this and other examples I conclude that a house or room often does symbolize a womb or a vagina in which the individual can escape in fantasy from the trials and anxieties of this life.

A peculiarity of the fantasy of prenatal regression is that in it there is sometimes represented, not only the blissful return to the mother, but also a reconciliation with the father. More often, perhaps, the father still appears as a possible disturber, as in the common dream in which the dreamer is in some dark and comfortable cavern but is all the time threatened by a mysterious monster outside who may be expected to penetrate at any moment. Sometimes, however, there is also a reconciliation with the monster, and this fantasy seems to underlie many of the conceptions of the other world. The dead Pharaoh was not only secure in his pyramid or rock-hewn grave and suckled by the goddess Nut or Isis,[1] but he also lived in blissful harmony with his father Re or Amon. This state is for the psycho-analyst reminiscent of certain dreams in which the fantasy of prenatal regression is combined with a feminine homosexual fantasy of union with the father. In such dreams

---

[1] Breasted, *Religion and Thought in Ancient Egypt*, 130, 137, 139.

the two incompatible desires of the Œdipus complex—namely the possession of the mother and the reconciliation with the father—are both attained and all the yearnings of a bisexual character are temporarily fulfilled.

The Trobriander spirit-world is known as Tuma. ' Every man, during his existence in Tuma, is able to rejuvenate from time to time, whenever he feels the burden of age. . . . Sometimes, however, the spirit goes back still further and becomes a diminutive being, a child just ready to enter a woman's body and to be born after a time.'[1] In primitive mythology, the place to which men return in death is often also the place from which the spirit children come, and this suggests that the theory of the last paragraph is not so fanciful as it may appear. Some day, perhaps, it may be possible to deduce psycho-analytic propositions from general biology or even from physiology, but at present conviction can only be obtained by those who have themselves been analysed. We can argue that much in mythology, in architecture, in sculpture, and in painting owes its origin and its appeal to certain unconscious fantasies, but we cannot yet hope to bring conviction.

212. *The incest drama.*

The unconscious factors involved in the production of romance are much more evident than those involved in the plastic arts. Otto Rank has devoted a great book to the subject and has shown how often a poem or legend is a thinly disguised incest fantasy.[2]

[1] Malinowski, ' Spirit Hunting in the South Seas,' *The Realist*, ii.

[2] *Das Inzest-Motiv.*

After the taboo on parricide and its extension to the murder of kinsmen, the taboo on incest is probably the earliest inhibition of mankind; for these were the taboos which made possible the development of the family into the clan. But no sooner had man repressed his incestuous tendencies than they began to find a distorted expression in myth, legend, and drama. First he projected openly upon his gods the tendencies which he had forbidden himself. So arose those myths of incestuous gods who married their mothers or their sisters.

In nearly all the Asiatic religions of which we have any record there is a myth of a Great Mother Goddess and her slain consort, who was either her brother or her son. Thus Attis, according to some accounts[1] was the son as well as the consort of Cybele. The classical example of son-mother incest in legend is the story of Œdipus. In more modern literature the same motive recurs in a disguised form as an intrigue between son and step-mother. Schiller's drama *Don Carlos*[2] is a good example of this variant of the incest fantasy.

213. *The tragic drama.*

A type of incest drama may be distinguished in which the hero, after attaining the summit of his ambition, does not live happily ever after but ends his career with a cataclysmic fall. This type of story may be called the tragic drama, and its clearest example is the legend of Œdipus who, after killing his father and possessing his

[1] Frazer, *Golden Bough*, 3rd ed., i, 263.
[2] See Rank, *Das Inzest-Motiv*, 56 ff.

mother, and her kingdom, is pursued by ill fortune and ends by tearing out his eyes. Such a story includes at once the summit of incestuous ambition with the most appalling punishment for this crime. The fascination of this story raises a severe problem for the hedonist, for it suggests to him that the craving for tragedy in fantasy may correspond to a craving for the real experience, and that real tragedy, however accidental it may seem, is sometimes self-inflicted.

Reik, especially, has attempted to deal with this problem. He, like other observers, has noticed a very persistent demand for punishment in man which is sometimes openly expressed by those who make false confessions of crimes solely in order to be punished. More often, however, the punishment is enjoyed vicariously in witnessing the religious sacrifice or legal punishment of others, or in sympathy with the hero of an heroic tragedy in drama. This demand for punishment is due to the inversion of aggressive tendencies which are often masochistically tinged by the inversion of sexual tendencies as well. In its simplest form it is a common reaction to the Œdipus complex. Because of a love for the father, the sexual jealousy and parricidal wishes are repressed, but they continue unconsciously and are projected. Sometimes they are still directed to their original object, as in the obsessional neurotic who is tormented by the fear lest some damage shall happen to his father from an unknown source. But, often, they are inverted against the subject himself. He may then live in great and irrational fear of God, of the law, of public opinion, or of his conscience, because he fears what is in reality his own projected and inverted hate. Sometimes the strain of fighting this impulse will be too great and he will commit a crime in order to be punished, confess an imaginary crime, or merely inflict an injury upon himself. Many of those who are, for no apparent reason, failures in life, have unconsciously brought this failure upon themselves in order to satisfy the need for punishment and their projected and inverted hate. This kind of neurotic incompetence is probably commoner to-day than it has been in the past ; for in earlier periods of history the need was recognized and catered for. The medieval church provided penances which were always in great demand, and even Sir Thomas More wore a hair shirt and kept a whip with which to beat himself.[1] When he was beheaded for an offence of which he was innocent, he embraced his executioner and welcomed his fate with a resignation which would have been impossible if it had not satisfied a demand for punishment. In fact an over-punctilious conscience seems to have been used deliberately to secure this end.

Men of other ages did not depend only upon their own penances and executions for the satisfaction of their inverted aggressiveness, for it was always possible to enjoy these things vicariously. There were burnings, beheadings, hangings, floggings, and pilloryings always to be seen, and the victims were usually expected to address the crowd and proclaim their guilt so that the spectators could fully enter into their feelings and expiate by proxy their own sense of sin.

To-day there are no such easy forms of gratification

[1] Froude, *History of England.*

for this impulse, and for those who have not acquired some sado-masochistic perversion there remains only the tragic drama or novel to satisfy their need for direct or vicarious misfortune. Possibly the need itself is less, but certainly a good deal of neurosis would not occur if there were still a more adequate provision for its satisfaction. Many of the so-called war neuroses were really post-war neuroses, and were due to the loss of dangers and discomforts which had become masochistic satisfactions. But with an increased knowledge of unconscious motives it is possible that the need will dwindle until it can find adequate outlet in that sense of duty which compels many to devote their lives to some form of social service rather than to pleasure. It may be remarked in passing that this kind of socially useful conscience, which is due to an unconscious sense of guilt, is especially found among those who have inherited wealth. It is a characteristic of men who, through no effort of their own, have found themselves better off than their fellows and have worked out their sense of guilt neither in a neurosis nor in a perversion but in a compulsion to social service. The socialist who relieves the leisured classes of this sense of guilt may also find that he has destroyed one of the main sources of disinterested work.

We must return from this digression to the evolution of the drama The tragic drama is generally supposed to have developed from the religious mystery and sacrifice.[1] Freud, in *Totem und Tabu*, was the first to point out the psycho-analytic importance of this develop-

[1] Reinach, *Cultes, Mythes et Religions*, ii, 100.

I

ment. In the rites and sacrifice of the totem animal who had become a son-god, that is, a god of vegetation who was sown in the earth and who thereby fertilized his mother the Earth-goddess, the primitive husbandmen relieved their own unconscious incestuous fantasies and vicariously expiated their guilt.[1] Such rites developed into the Greek tragedy with its hero and chorus who mourned his agony. At first there were no spectators, then these were admitted as a sort of lay addition to the chorus, and finally the chorus itself disappeared when the spectators had learnt through their example to follow the drama in emotion, but to follow it in silence.

214. *Art as a reaction to false threats.*

In some such way as this we must infer that all the arts have been developed as the symbolic expression of repressed desires. To the spectator they seem to satisfy previously undiscovered yearnings. But the psychologist must admit the possibility that some of the relief they provide may lie in the removal of false threats, or in the provision of inadequate means. The child may suck its thumb to remove the false threat of hunger, and the satisfaction of an erotic appetite in the absence of a real need is perhaps always of this nature. When there is real hunger the thumb does not bring lasting satisfaction. Similarly, the phallic or vaginal symbolism of a picture or a statue does not secure the real object that it symbolizes, nor does the incest or tragic drama give the real objects of desire. But in so far as the

---

[1] I have elaborated this theme further in my book *The Meaning of Sacrifice* (Hogarth Press).

desire for these objects is due to a false threat of aphanisis the satisfaction is complete. Artists need not fear that psycho-analysis, at least as we know it, will ever free us from such irrelevant or inadequate seekings.[1]

22. Magic.

Magic, we have seen, differs from art in that the symbolic activity which it involves is rationalized, but rationalized falsely. It has often been stated that magic preceded art and that art evolved from magic. Those who take this view have argued, for instance, that the cave drawings of primitive man, which are the earliest pictures known, must have had a magical purpose. In some drawings the animal is depicted with an arrow through it, and this representation, it is argued, must have been supposed to secure magically the corresponding fact.[2] It is difficult to decide this question of priority, but it seems most natural to believe that purely symbolic acts of art must have occurred before these acts were rationalized. The drama is assumed to have evolved from the magical rite, but there is no reason why the magical rite may not itself be derived from an unrationalized act of still more primitive drama.

221. Sacrificial magic.

It has been argued by Freud and others,[3] including

[1] Cf. Chap. vi.

[2] Sollas, Ancient Hunters, 2nd ed., 358 ff.

[3] Freud, Totem und Tabu; Reik, Probleme der Religions psychologie; Roheim, Australian Totemism; Animism, Magic, and the Divine King.

the present author[1] that the earliest sacrifices, which were sacrifices *of* a god or revered animal, were symbolic representations of repressed parricidal fantasies. Certainly in historic times such acts were rationalized as fertility or other rites, but it is plausible to suppose that they were once performed without any rationalization. The unconscious desire to kill the father was undoubtedly symbolically expressed in the ritual slaughter of an animal which was especially revered and regarded as the ancestor or elder brother of the clan. Thus the Arabs, according to Nilus, appear to have sacrificed a camel by tearing it to pieces and consuming it raw. Many authors (e.g. Reinach) think that such rites were once universal, though the motives for them which are given are very varied. Robertson Smith[2] regarded them as acts of communion in which the worshippers cemented their kinship with each other and with their god by eating him. Frazer supposes that, in the sacrifice, the spirit of a vegetation deity was transferred from an old representative to the body of a whole and hearty successor, and also that the rite secured the fertility of the soil. The variety of the explanations offered and the difficulty of extending existing explanations to new rites suggests that the sacrificers themselves often had no very clear conscious rationalization of their acts, and that, even where such conscious motives have been worked out by early theology, they were late additions to the rites.

If, then, this argument is correct, totemic sacrifice existed as a ritual satisfaction of unconscious parricidal

[1] *Op. cit., The Meaning of Sacrifice.*
[2] *The Religion of the Semites.*

tendencies long before magical or religious rationalizations were added. When there is no outlet for these tendencies they are apt to invert against the subject and provoke a state of pessimism and foreboding. We should expect the primitive man, whose repressed parricidal tendencies are strong, to be subject to such depression to a great extent, and this expectation is confirmed by the commonness of suicide and neurosis among primitive peoples. By killing a father symbol in sacrifice the primitive man can work off his aggressive tendencies and prevent them from turning upon himself. The subsequent reaction of elation and freedom from taboo which we should expect has been noted by many observers in the orgies which frequently follow the sacrifice. ' The occasions of religious ceremonial on which licence is allowed are at initiation ceremonies, at funerals, and at the feasts in honour of the " divinities. ' '1 Such organized licence may be compared with the ' ritual laugh.'2

Among primitive peoples, the elation of ritually killing an animal which was a father symbol might well produce a general optimism which would readily attach itself to any enterprise. And, since even the civilized individual can seldom adequately distinguish subjective from objective grounds for optimism, a rite which evoked elation might well come to be regarded as a rite which

1 Evans-Pritchard, ' Some Collective Expressions of Obscenity in Africa,' *Journal of the Royal Anthropological Institute*, lix, 313.

2 ' Les Sardes riaient en sacrifiant leurs vieillards; les Troglodytes, en lapidant leurs morts ; les Phéniciens, quand on immolait leurs enfants ; les Thraces, quand l'un d'eux venait à mourir.' Reinach, *Cultes, Mythes et Religions*, iv, 124.

secured success. The conscious rationalization of sacrifice would naturally vary according to the occupations of the sacrificers. Hunters would believe that it secured their prey, herdsmen that it promoted the fertility of their flocks, agriculturists that it secured abundant harvest, and warriors that it guaranteed their victory. Once the supposed causal association had been established, the rite would be varied to correspond more closely with the end desired.

At a later stage such actions were no longer supposed to operate automatically, but only through the agency of some spirit, so that the simple magical rite, in so far as it survived, had to be re-rationalized as a religious rite. The definition we have given of a magical act as a falsely rationalized symbolic act really covers a great deal of what is usually relegated to religion, for a religious rite is often also a symbolic act which is falsely rationalized. The difference depends upon whether or not the rationalization involves the intervention of an imaginary supernatural being We may distinguish the two sorts of magic by qualifying them respectively as non-religious or as religious.

A sacrificial rite passed from the domain of non-religious magic to that of religious magic when it was reinterpreted as a communion, an expiation, a gift, or a homage. The unconscious motive which it satisfied was probably still some distorted form of parricide,[1] but the rationalization was different. In the communal sacrifice the rationalized intention was to cement or re-cement the kinship between the worshippers and

[1] *Op. cit., The Meaning of Sacrifice.*

their god.[1] In the expiatory, or gift, sacrifice the god, who was originally the victim, became the recipient, and the consciously anticipated result, even if it remained the same successful enterprise, was believed to be secured by the intervention of this god. But often the expected result was immateralized into forgiveness ; and in the homage sacrifice no result whatever was anticipated, the rite being interpreted as an appropriate gesture on the part of the worshipper which was itself its own reward.

In sacrifices in which the victim became the god's son the older idea of communion survived to complicate the later idea of expiation. Frazer[2] has collected many examples of this kind of rite, which may be illustrated in the cults of Attis, Adonis, and Orpheus, and has survived in the Christian Eucharist. Since the worshippers ate their god, the sacrifice was communal, and since they identified themselves with him it was also expiatory. But traces of a magical purpose still survive. The rites were associated with sowing or reaping and were believed to stimulate the crops.

222. *Other forms of magic.*

There are of course many other forms of magic besides those we find in sacrifice. But I think that it can be shown that they all result from the rationalization of some action which satisfies symbolically an unconscious desire. One may first distinguish between public and private magic, between magic authorized by tradition

[1] Robertson Smith, *The Religion of the Semites.*
[2] *The Golden Bough.*

and handed down to the whole community, and magic practised by the professional magician ; but, since the unconscious motives involved in both forms are of the same kind, it is unnecessary to elaborate this distinction here. For the purpose of this study the best classification would be according to the unconscious motive. In sacrifice I believe that the main unconscious motive is nearly always parricide.

The results of psycho-analysis should suggest to us that, wherever unconscious parricidal tendencies are found incestuous desires cannot be far away, for the incest wish is the motive of parricidal jealousy. Associated with the sacrifice of the great Asiatic gods of fertility there is often a representation of the marriage between the god and his consort, who is often his mother or his sister. Thus Dionysus was annually married to the queen of Athens.[1] Such customs were world-wide and were intended to stimulate the fertility of the soil. They appear to have symbolized an incestuous union between the god of vegetation and his mother the Earth. An unauthorised incest was generally supposed to have exactly the opposite effect, and to blight the crops. But, in the religious festival, each participant could vicariously enjoy at once the crime and punishment by identifying himself with his god. Since the earth was already a symbol of the mother such rites could be easily rationalized as aids to agriculture, for to fertilize the mother was to fertilize the earth.

There is a very common type of private magic in which an image is made of some enemy, and the

---

[1] Frazer, *Golden Bough*, ii, 136 ff. ; vii, 30 ff.

injury inflicted upon the model is believed to operate against the original. In such practices the unconscious motive is very much the same as the conscious one, but the belief in their efficacy probably depends upon the satisfaction given to an unconscious which knows no difference between sensations and ideas.

Similar in method but different in aim to the magical injury of an enemy is the magical process by which the love of an adored individual is secured. An image is made, containing if possible some object which has been in contact with its original, and pierced to the heart or otherwise operated upon in a suitable manner.[1] Such practices are believed infallible. The conscious and unconscious motives are again similar, though the belief in the efficacy of the operation probably depends upon the credulity of the unconscious. In the older rites the attack was perhaps directed with less delicacy to an organ of the body other than the heart, and to the unconscious the more indirect approach of the later practice probably retains its original meaning.

In passing we may note that the similarity between rites to kill an enemy and to secure a wife[2] is further evidence of the phylogenetic derivation of the aggressive impulse from the sexual impulse.[3]

More interesting and more obscure than these last two types of magic are types in which security from

---

[1] See Frazer, *Golden Bough*, 3rd ed., i, 77.

[2] This similarity forms the main theme in Dumas' novel, *La Reine Margot*.

[3] *Cf.* Chap. iii, 2252.

some evil influence is obtained by a magic circle. Thus, a town may be surrounded by a furrow, an individual may be made to pass through the corpse of an animal, or an army may be marched between the two halves of a victim. Such rites are reminiscent of ceremonies of rebirth in which the novice is made to crawl between the legs of his mother. But they are also reminiscent of the fantasy of prenatal regression which is acted in the burial rites of so many peoples. Possibly the relief they bring is due to their symbolizing an escape to the mother from the father, and the satisfaction of the incestuous desire, i.e. an escape from the false threats which the child has never outgrown.

Another favourite method of warding off evil was to wear some talisman, usually a phallic symbol. Indeed the earliest talismans were often simple representations of the male organ, so that here again history helps to confirm the psycho-analytic interpretation. The evil fortune which was avoided in this way was at first generally impotence or sterility, and the same recipe seems to have been later applied to guard against ill fortune of almost any kind. Needless to say, it was the false threat of sterility rather than the real evil which was avoided in this manner. The display of the symbol reassured the unconscious that its castrating impulse, which had been projected and inverted, had not yet attained its object. For in the unconscious there is no distinction between idea and sensation, or desire and fact, and the idea of the loss of the penis, evoked by the inverted desire, can only be countered by the idea of its possession evoked by the symbolic talisman. The embarrasment and loss of self-confidence which may sometimes be observed to-day in the man who drops his stick or his monocle, or who suddenly finds himself without his tie, shows that such symbolic objects still operate as phallic talismans.

23. *Science.*

We have defined science as a symbolic activity with a true rationalization. In other words, science is an activity which fulfils both unconscious and conscious motives. In art there is no utilitarian motive, in magic the utilitarian motive is falsely believed to be satisfied, but in science the secondary motive is really fulfilled. This view of science is in direct opposition to that expressed in the dictum ' necessity is the mother of invention.' In rare cases the sole motive for scientific discovery may have been practical necessity alone, but far more often science springs from an obsessional compulsion to create contrivances or theories which symbolize something desired by the unconscious and which have only a secondary practical utility.

It has often been said that science developed out of magic,[1] but it would seem equally true to assert that it had developed from art. For science is separated into two divisions, the pure and the applied ; and while it is true that the applied branch of science is derived from magic, it would seem more correct to regard the pure branch as a development from art. It has also been said that pure science is derived from applied science,

[1] Frazer, *Golden Bough*, i, 219; xi, 304 ff. Reinach, *Cultes, Mythes et Religions*, iii, 106.

but the two branches appear to have had largely independent origins, the one purely speculative from art through astrology to astronomy, philosophy, and physics, the other purely practical from magic through medicine to physiology and chemistry. But such schemes of development must not be taken too seriously, for the categories of art, magic, and pure and applied science are not mutually exclusive. And even if these categories did not overlap, the derivation of pure science from art, and applied science from magic, is only a rough generalization to which there are exceptions. The applied science of mechanics contributed to the concepts of pure physics.

231. *From astrology to physics.*

Art was seldom purely imitative ; for man introduced into his model a design which was not in the original, but which symbolized an object of unconscious desire. Thus the composition of early pictures often contains, as we have seen, phallic and vaginal symbols which perhaps still constitute part of their appeal. If man distorted the things which he could see, there was a much greater scope for this tendency when he attempted to represent the things which he could not see. The earliest representations of the universe in legend or in relief disclose the product of an unconscious fantasy almost wholly unchecked by real knowledge of the object portrayed. To primitive man the great vault of the sky was a solid or liquid sphere on which the sun-god drove his chariot or was rowed in a boat. Rank has argued that such theories were products of the unconscious fantasy of pre-natal regression,[1] and some confirmation of this view may be found in the Egyptian concept of the sky-goddess Nut, in whose womb the dead Pharaoh rested as the sun-god Re.

Only gradually was the free play of fantasy limited by real observation. And even now it is a mistake to suppose that theories are worked out in order to fit facts. The observation of facts never has provided, and perhaps never will provide, the real motive for the construction of theories ; but observation may determine which theories will be selected. Anyone with introspective ability, who has done research work, would probably admit that this was so ; for, if he considered the matter, he would find that he suffered from the artist's compulsion to produce intellectual structures, and that the one-one correlation with facts, which some of them afterwards are found to possess, was not the aim of his work, but a welcome justification of what might otherwise have been an idle pleasure.

It was many centuries before the early metaphysician deigned to test his elegant conceptions by comparing them with facts. And even then he did not scrap them altogether, but only modified them and selected those modifications which seemed to have the closest relation with observation. The vault of heaven was multiplied into several spheres which carried the sun, the fixed stars, and the planets. But the earth, in the centre of these spheres, still resembled the child in the womb and suggested the comforting security which this fantasy was invented to provide.

[1] *The Trauma of Birth.*

Galileo had the courage to vacate this position in favour of the sun, but the storm which he thereby evoked was due to the destruction of a fantasy which operated like a talisman. His contemporaries felt that the acceptance of his theory was equivalent to a second banishment from Eden, and they fought tenaciously against it. Perhaps the scientist must always have an element of sado-masochism in his make-up before he can deprive others, as well as himself, of some cherished superstition.

Parallel with the destruction of the egocentric conception of the universe was the destruction of its soul. At first man projected his own impulses upon those relatively stable complexes of sensation which he called objects,[1] and regarded all nature as animate, subject to good and bad intentions like himself. Later he separated distinct personalities from objects and thought of them no longer as themselves animate, but as controlled each by its own peculiar spirit. The next stage was to promote the spirits of certain important objects, such as the sun, the moon, the rivers, or the vegetation, to a high position as rulers of all other things—a stage which began in the monotheism of the speculative Akhnaton and culminated in the theology of the omnipotent God of Jewish theology. Gradually, however, science stripped objects of their animistic attributes, until it not only deprived them of their independent wills but also removed them from the direct intervention of their supposed creator. Projected muscular sensibility was the last to go, and, even to the present day, the concept of force and

[1] Mach, *Analyse der Empfindungen.*

substance has not been completely banished. But the culture of a future age will doubtless look upon the materialistic physics of the beginning of this century as we do upon the still more blatant animistic conceptions of our predecessors.[1]

232. From magic to chemistry.

Roheim, in the course of a stimulating paper,[2] outlines the development from black magic, through white magic, to the scientific medicine of to-day.

We have seen how the super-ego is formed by the introjection of a concept of the father which was originally formed by the projection of the subject's own aggressive tendencies, and how, ever after, it remains as a largely unconscious conscience which represses many of the aggressive and sexual impulses.[3] But these impulses remain in the unconscious and find distorted outlets either in sublimations or in perversions. The sublimations are new activities which seek something which symbolizes what is forbidden, but the perversions are only new editions of old pre-genital activities which would otherwise have been replaced by the repressed genital impulses. If the pre-genital perversions are also repressed they will give rise either to further sublimations or to neuroses.

Roheim, following Freud,[4] argues that in primeval

[1] Cf. Chap. ii.
[2] " Nach dem Tode des Urvaters ", Imago, ix. An abstract of this paper by the present author appears in the British Journal of Medical Psychology, ix.
[3] Cf. Chap. iv, 15.
[4] Totem und Tabu.

days, exiled herds of tribal brothers used to break in upon their family and kill and eat their father, believing, like all cannibals, that they absorbed his character with his body. They thus introjected him physically as well as mentally, and Roheim argues that the act of eating reinforced the psychic identification. After this, the enemy was no longer in the outer world, but a part of the subject himself whom he could no longer attack, except by suicide ; from whom he could no longer escape, and by whom he felt himself possessed. It was this introjection, according to Roheim, which first caused the repression of genital impulses expressed in the incest and endogamic taboos and diverted them to the sublimations of culture and the regressions of perversion and neurosis.

Among the brothers who thus ate their father there would be dispositional differences, and among those who in virtue of their innate qualities regressed permanently to the anal erotic level, Roheim believes that he detects the first black magicians and the cultural ancestors of the doctors of to-day. The black magician, he points out, is fundamentally an anal erotic pervert, but a pervert who believes that his acts fulfil a real purpose. Thus, the magician's typical procedure is to procure a sample of the excrement of his enemy and burn it, after which he believes that his victim will surely die.

The medicine man, who cures rather than kills, Roheim derives from the black magician who has repressed and sublimated his anal-sadistic impulses. It is not difficult to show that the medicine man's magic is in fact an anal sublimation. The chief magical instrument of the Australian shaman, which he uses to cure his clients as well as to injure their enemies, is the quartz crystal. That this crystal is really an excrement symbol is clearly shown by the beliefs which surround it, and we may further conjecture that it symbolizes the excrement of the father and that it owes its supposed power to this fact. It is believed that the shaman keeps it in his intestines or in his stomach, and that it and a new set of intestines is given him by the ancestral spirits. Some of the Australian tribes say that it is the excrement of the Sky-God, and West Australians believe that the analogous magical stuff *boglia* is acquired at the death of the father, and that it is derived from the human body, especially the anus.[1]

Similar practices from other parts of the world could no doubt be cited to illustrate the pre-history of medicine. For many centuries the medicine man held in the estimation of his fellows an almost divine position, and, as a father symbol, was long exalted above criticism. But this very position attracted to him inevitably a large element of unconscious hate, which, when the solidarity of medico-priestly superstition was weakened by the contact of rival cultures, was not long in expressing itself at first as doubt and then as open criticism. The medicine man was forced to discard his useless practices and to discover new ones. But his investigations were still motivated by unconscious impulses, and his new methods did not at first differ from the old in that they were less the sublimates of anal-sadistic tendencies, but only in that they were more carefully selected. The

[1] Roheim, *Ib.*, 101.

K

function of the unconscious was still to create, that of observation was employed, then as now, only to eliminate what was practically useless. The first genuine medicine which was discovered was probably the purgative.

The further development of medicine loses itself in a maze of complexity too great to be followed here, but a painstaking psycho-analyst could doubtless show that many of its advances were due to these same two forces of unconscious creation and conscious selection. I do not suggest that anal-sadistic sublimations are the only factors in early medicine, but only that they are the easiest factors to abstract. This essay is intended only to illustrate the method of development, and not to follow it in detail.

The historical parents of the chemist of to-day were the herbalist and the alchemist. The former in his search for effective purgatives, and the latter in his quest for something which would turn everything into gold, which is a well established excrement symbol,[1] again illustrate the unconscious anal interest which determines these activities.

233. *From architecture to mechanics.*

The development from art to architecture, from architecture to mechanics, and from mechanics to physics, forms an exception to a more general rule.

---

[1] Ernest Jones, *Psycho-Analysis*, 2nd ed., 1918, 676-8. Seligman reports a case of an insane native of Suau (Massim) who asserted that his faeces were money, "Temperament, Conflict and Psychosis in a Stone-Age Population," *British Journal of Medical Psychology*, ix, 196.

For while the pure sciences seem usually to have evolved from art, and the applied sciences from magic, the applied science of mechanics seems to have been mainly derived from an art—though an art which borders on magic—and to have become one of the ancestors of the purest science.

Architecture, we have seen reason to believe, owed its origin to no practical need, but to man's unconscious desire to return in death to the womb from which he came. He began to create for himself tombs in the image of the object he wished to inhabit, and to cause himself to be buried in the uterine position. But soon such customs were rationalized as magical rites to secure immortality.

The temple evolved from the tomb and the house from the temple, and, as we have seen, these later structures often still possess the same symbolic meaning. But building necessitated a knowledge of mechanics, so that one root of this science was derived from architecture.

There was, however, another source of mechanics in the cosmogonies of early speculation, and this root flourished for a long time unsullied by any practical application. These two divisions roughly correspond to statics and dynamics, and, while the former seems always to have been associated with the concrete problems of building, the latter was for a long time purely speculative.

Both divisions of mechanics, however, have this in common, that they involve a projection of muscular sensibility into those relatively stable complexes of sensation which are called objects. How far this projection is a relic of animism it is difficult to say. Probably animals who have never formed the concept of ghosts or spirits nevertheless associate tactual memories with seen objects, especially when two such objects are seen to collide.[1] But there is no doubt that the animism which is due to the projection of repressed aggressiveness, has always played, and still plays, a great part in the conceptions of force, causality, and law.

Our present conception of the universe is largely mechanistic, and it is still difficult for us to realize that this is a projection of our own muscular and tactual impulses. But we may remember that the theological cosmogony of our ancestors must have seemed as self-evident to them as the mechanistic and material universe does to us. We now recognize the animistic and spiritualistic conceptions of the past to be but anthropomorphic projections. The dullest of our descendants, enjoying an understanding as penetrating as that of Hume, will regard our own material universe with more tolerance for the errors of a bygone age, but with no less contempt.

[1] Money-Kyrle, "Belief and Representation," *Symposion* i ; see also Chap. i.

CHAPTER V

THE ONTOGENESIS OF IMPULSES

I. *The relation between ontogenesis and phylogenesis.*
II. *Emergent instincts.*

THERE is a certain analogy between the execution of a series of post-hypnotic suggestions and the development of the impulses of man. To the individual who has awakened from hypnotic sleep his acts seem but the natural consequences of former conscious motives, and it is difficult to convince him that they are really due to unconscious suggestions. To the child his new impulses seem to be intelligent developments of the old, rather than consequences of innate dispositions. In both cases conscious motives are selected which satisfy also the predetermined purpose. In the following discussion we shall be in danger of the same error as the subject of hypnosis or the child. The development of impulses from one another will sometimes seem the inevitable action of environment upon a fortuitous collection of receptors, nerve fibres, and effectors devoid of pre-determined pattern. But when we are tempted to think thus, we should remember the hypnotic suggestion. New impulses are developed, not because they are the only possible modifications of the old, but because they are the only ones, from innumerable possibilities, which correspond to inborn dispositions. The individual finds his way, not because it is the only way, but because the race has blazed the trail.

12. *The theory of recapitulation.*

It is a working theory of biology that ontogenesis is a recapitulation of phylogenesis. The individual, it is assumed, develops the same characteristics in the same order as the race, and this theory helps us to transfer the knowledge we gain in one science to the other. When we discover anything about the individual it suggests a parallel for investigation in the race, or when we discover anything about the race it compels us to look for similarities in the individual. Further, the theory has a negative as well as a positive value. It saves us from error as well as leading us to truth. For it makes us suspicious of any supposed development of the individual which is not reflected in the race, or of the race which is not reflected in the individual.

But useful as the theory of recapitulation often is, it is also sometimes misleading, since it is only an approximation to the truth. Each individual of the race has blazed a certain trail from his origin as a single cell to his end in death. This trail leaves (Lamarck), or results from (Darwin), a disposition which is transmitted. If the theory of recapitulation were exactly true, the descendant might prolong the road taken by his ancestor, but he could not otherwise improve it. But we know that the individual not only extends the trail, but that he also takes short cuts.

This caution may serve to anticipate a criticism of certain parts of the discussion of this section. We shall describe a theory of the development of the sexual impulse which can only be applied to mammals. Since coitus is an older biological invention than breast feeding, this development cannot be a close recapitulation of the history of the race. But man may have made short cuts which were unknown to his pre-mammalian ancestors.

2. *The biography of the soma.*

After this warning I will try to systematize briefly what psycho-analysis has discovered or suggested about the growth of the higher interests of man from the simple needs of the skin, the stomach, the bowels, the kidneys, and the glands of sex. The attempt may not be successful, but, since in nature there are no discontinuities and the complex is a derivative of the simple, it is justified in principle.

21. *Birth-trauma and pre-natal regression.*

The child, before his birth, is almost completely protected from injuries or needs. The outside world cannot hurt him, nor can he feel suffocation or hunger as long as his blood vessels are continuous with those of his mother. From his tranquil sleep he is suddenly awakened by the discomfort of the act of birth and by the sensations of cold and suffocation. Soon he learns to breathe, is put in a warm and comfortable place, and goes to sleep. But we might expect him to have acquired a sense of insecurity which will never leave him till his death. In particular, we might expect that slight experiences of cold, pain, or suffocation would act as threats which recall the shock of birth.

There is some psycho-analytical evidence that situations which are associated with, or which symbolize, the event of birth do evoke anxiety. The cause of claustrophobia, for instance, may be partly an association of the idea of being in a confined space with a dim memory of the shock of birth. But, although it is plausible to suppose that the shock of birth may persist into later life, it seems extravagant to derive, as Rank does,[1] every anxiety from this event. Apart from other possible objections to this extreme form of the theory, it is at least unlikely that fear, which appears to be common to every zoological species, in man is derived from an experience which he only shares with other viviparous mammals. It is thus not safe to go beyond the vague statement that the memory of the shock of birth is an element in all subsequent experiences of fear.[2]

Some psycho-analysts believe not only in a fear of a repetition of the shock of birth but also in a desire to return to the pre-natal condition. Rank and Ferenczi, again adopting an extreme view, have attempted to derive all the impulses of man from this supposed urge. According to them the child always seeks the womb which he dimly remembers as the means to the removal of all his subsequent injuries and needs. They see in the history of his impulses an ever more perfect realization of this old means, from the time when he feeds upon

---

[1] Op. cit., The Trauma of Birth.
[2] Freud, Vorlesungen, 4th ed., 461.

his mother's milk till he attains a symbolically complete return in the act of coitus.[1]

This theory has the merit of giving an organic foundation to that unconscious tendency to incest which psycho-analysis and psycho-analytical anthropology agree in regarding as universal. But, like the extreme form of the theory of the shock of birth, it has the defect that it is only applicable to the higher mammals. The cock's impulse to penetrate the hen can scarcely be derived from his desire to return to the egg. Thus, if coitus in the higher animals is due to an urge to return to the pre-natal state, ontogenesis must have made short cuts which phylogenesis did not take.

The theory of the birth trauma and of the urge to pre-natal regression both derive their support from the same class of facts. In the dreams of the civilized, and in the myths and rites of primitive peoples,[2] a fantasy of pre-natal life is often represented. Sometimes such fantasies are associated with anxiety and sometimes with longing, and these two types are quoted respectively in support of the theory of the birth trauma and of a fundamental desire for pre-natal regression. But, as has been pointed out by Freud, the same two fantasies may equally symbolize a coitus, in which a part is represented by a whole, and which may be associated either with anxiety or desire. Therefore the empirical evidence of both theories is ambiguous.

There are biological objections to the extreme form

[1] Rank, Op, cit., The Trauma of Birth; Ferenczi, Versuch einer Genitaltheorie.
[2] Cf. Chap. iv, 21.

of both theories. But we may believe in the persistence of the shock of birth or in the desire for pre-natal regression without promoting either tendency to a supreme position as the origin of all fear or all desire.

22. Oral impulses.

After the need for air, perhaps the most primitive part of the need rhythm proceeds from the organism's periodic lack of food. On such occasions certain internal stimuli occur which evoke central processes correlated with the unpleasure of hunger. This is at first followed by random movements, if the crying and fidgetting of the new-born babe is entirely random. At this stage, in so far as desires are imperfectly innate, there is no clear idea of milk or of the sensations of drinking. Soon, however, after the child has enjoyed the experience of being fed, we must suppose that the random reactions give place to seekings, and the dim unpleasure to the specific desire. This desire, we have supposed,[1] is made up of the sensation of the need, that is, the hunger plus the idea of the means, that is, the mother's breasts. Then, if the seeking, that is, the purposeful cry, is successful and the breasts arrive, the combined stimuli of need and means evoke the final removal. Parallel with these physical events, want gives way to desire, desire to appetite, and appetite to the partial death of satiation. Thus, after the child has had a few experiences of feeding, the want or unpleasure of hunger will expand into the desire, which includes an image of the breasts, and the desire into the

[1] Cf. Chap. ii, 2.

appetite which anticipates the sensations accompanying removal.

It is, however, not only a need that can provoke desire, but also the threat of a need. Loneliness, and darkness, which is interpreted as loneliness, are a real terror to the child, and I believe that this terror is largely the fear of hunger.[1] Hunger is one of the first experiences of the child, and it is difficult for the civilized and comfortable individual to imagine what this can mean to one who has not yet learnt to rely on the certainty of his next meal. But the Egyptians, who dwelt on the borders of the desert, had not forgotten. The texts of the Book of the Dead, which comfort the dying king by the promise of the ' pendent breasts ' of his divine mother[2], prove that their fears were survivals of infancy, preserved, rather than created, by the conditions under which they lived.

A fear is the sensation of a threat plus the idea of an injury or need. And, if I am right in supposing that loneliness is to the child a threat of hunger, the fear of loneliness must include the unpleasure of imagined hunger. It is well known that fear is often accompanied by sensations of hunger, and this may be because the fear is partly derived from the hunger anxiety of the lonely child. The fact that the child's fear gives rise to the same desire for the mother as the unpleasure of hunger seems further to confirm this view.

But the mother cannot be always with the child, so that he must learn to do without her. When he is

---

[1] *Cf.* Chap. ii, 121 ; Chap. iii, 221.
[2] Breasted, *Religion and Thought in Ancient Egypt*, 130, 137, 139.

lonely and afraid, he sucks his thumb, and, since his desire to do so is not due to a real need but to a false threat, this substitute for the real means may remove his fear. Moreover, since the thumb stimulates the lips, it evokes a partial appetite which is the more pleasurable because it is unsullied by the sensation of a real need. Such a partial appetite perhaps forms the basis of those oral erotic sensations, which are later enriched by associations with true genital eroticism.

The thumb thus becomes a solace and the instrument of a pleasure. To the criminal the hardest deprivation of prison life is to be denied tobacco ; for the pipe, which would cheer him in his solitude, is the lineal descendant of the thumb which once robbed loneliness of the threat of hunger. The real oral needs of the civilized individual are easily satisfied. But the threat of these needs, which he experienced in infancy, may survive as the fear of loneliness, or of darkness and death, which are forms of loneliness. The thumb, which was the fictitious means to the removal of a false threat, lives on in some new form to help to still these fears.

Other oral impulses, such as those of kissing, fellatio, or coprophagia, are more obviously mixed with impulses from different spheres and will be considered later.

Psycho-anaylsts have divided the oral stage of libidinal development into two sub-stages. In the first sub-stage the object of the impulse is loved ; in the second it is also hated. What exactly makes up this love it is difficult to say, but the child has a sort of yearning for the breasts, the comforter, or the thumb, which seems to be a mixture of desire and fear, desire for the object and fear lest it should be lost. It is perhaps this uncertainty of possession which makes up the sorrow which may often be detected in love.

It is still more difficult to analyse the hate which complicates the love in the second oral stage. It is comparable to the attitude of a young tiger which was described as munching a bone as if he hated it, and I have seen kittens behave in the same ominous way the first time they were given a rat to eat. There is no doubt that every child has something of the carnivore about him, and that the cannibalistic interest of his games is more deep-seated than the adult and civilized observer would care to own. Therefore, when little boys at a certain age persistently play at eating or being eaten by their parents, we may infer that a similar, but more earnest, wish is present in the unconscious.

Hate, like love, pursues its object, and is expressed by set teeth and grinding jaw. Thus part of its aim is to eat the object, which is also the aim of oral love. It has often been said that anger is the child of fear, and hate the offspring of thwarted love. The first interference does not come from a rival but from the mother herself. Therefore it would seem that the child who bites his mother in the second oral phase acts in the frenzy of his first great disappointment.

Freud, in his later works,[1] regards the love and death impulses as the two fundamental urges of life. But, whereas love satisfies a definite physiological need, it is

[1] *Das Unbehagen in der Kultur, Jenseits des Lustprinzips.*

difficult to imagine what analogous chemical substances there can be, which accumulate and stimulate and can only be excreted by an act of hate. Freud's insight has been proved to be extraordinarily acute, and it is possible that such substances exist as the physiological consequences of his theory seem to require.[1] But for the moment, it seems more plausible to regard the hate as a reaction to the frustration of any impulse, especially the oral and the sexual, than as an independent primordial urge.

We may perhaps point out in passing that the development of hate may be another exception to the theory of recapitulation. We have seen reason to believe that, phylogenetically, hate originated as a by-product of the sexual impulse, and that the weapons of male animals were first evolved to master the female before they were applied to defeat rivals. But, ontogenetically, hate is a by-product of the oral impulse. Aggressiveness, which was originally evolved to master the female, must have been taken over by, and adapted to, oral impulses in carnivores, so that ontogenesis exhibits the development of the derivative before the impulse from which it was derived.

23. Anal impulses.

After the oral erotic stage of development, analysts distinguish an anal stage, which is again sub-divided. The first sub-stage is characterized by a great pleasure in defecating and the second by an obstinate refusal to do so to please others. Thus the dirtiness of the baby

---

[1] See Chap. iii, 225.

is followed by the apparent constipation of the child. It seems probable that anal erotic sensations are developed very much in the same way as oral erotic sensations, though since there is at first no necessity for an external means and no seeking to be learnt, the process must be shorter. The anal need and unpleasure probably give rise at first to quite random movements, until the correct removal is learnt. The sensations which accompany the process of defecation, like the sensations of drinking, help to sustain the act. The memory of these sensations is evoked by the need, and the unpleasure develops into the desire or appetite, which is made up of the sensation of the need plus the idea of the sensations which will accompany its removal.

Just as there develops a fictitious oral appetite apart from an oral need, so there seems to arise a fictitious anal appetite apart from an anal need. Thus, to the phenomenon of thumb sucking, there corresponds anal masturbation. But anal, even more than oral, eroticism seems to be derived from associations with true genital sensations.

We have seen that anal impulses, unlike oral impulses, are originally objectless. That is, the final removal does not necessitate the presence of a means. But, under the conditions of civilization, the child is soon taught not to relieve himself as and when he will. He must first call for his nurse or mother to attend to him. Thus a seeking reaction is artificially interposed between the need and its removal. This fact may possibly facilitate that sexualization of anal impulses

which appears to be more developed in the perversions of civilized peoples than in those of
savages.[1]

We know from analysis that the act of defecation
is for the child an act of love, and that he will perform
it only for those he loves. We know, further, that
the products are regarded as articles of value. It seems
probable that the attribution of value to the faeces,
and the conception of their surrender as an act of
love are mainly the result of oral contributions to the
anal impulse. We know from analysis that the buttocks
are often symbols of the breasts, and it seems likely
that when the child discovers his own buttocks he
treats them as substitutes for his mother's breasts
and values them accordingly.[2] They become a fictitious means to still the old but ever present threat
of loneliness and hunger, or aphanisis as Ernest Jones
would say. From this it follows that children are
liable to pass through a coprophagic stage, in which
they desire consciously or unconsciously to eat their
own faeces as substitutes for the milk which is now
denied them. I have heard children say that ' big
business is delicious,' and all analysts must have come
across similar infantile survivals in their patients.
The Egyptian of the time of the pyramids was terrified
lest he should be forced by hunger in the next world
to eat his own excrement,[3] and it would seem that the
fear is the conscious reaction to the infantile uncon-

---

[1] Malinowski, *The Sexual Life of Savages*, 395 ff.
[2] See Chap. iii, 222.
[3] Breasted, *Religion and Thought in Ancient Egypt*, 130, 282.

scious wish. If the goddess Nut does not take pity upon him and feed him from her 'pendent breasts,'[1] he has at least a substitute in the products of his own buttocks.[2]

It is perhaps at this stage, in which oral impulses are symbolically satisfied in anal fantasies, that the child first begins to project his own impulses upon others. In the unconscious anal fantasy of eating the product of his own buttocks he learns to play the roles of both receiving and giving. And, in so far as he dimly remembers his mother's act of giving milk, he conceives of it in terms of his own act of giving faeces.[3] He projects his sensations of giving or letting go, to help to build up his idea of the mother who gives him his nourishment from her own body. This idea is very tender and not at all disgusting to the child, and it is not so far from the truth as first appears. For his mother, in her own infancy, formed a similar idea of the sensation of giving suck, and this idea survives unconsciously to complicate the actual sensation[4]. It may be disturbing, but it is none the less true, that much of our most deep and tender feeling is

[1] *Ib.* 130, 137, 139.

[2] Analysts tell us that machines to secure perpetual motion owe much of the impulse of their creation to similar infantile fantasies.

[3] The child at first has no disgust, and all bodily excretions are liable to become associated with milk and valued accordingly.

[4] The unconscious association between milk and faeces was doubtless responsible for the accusation sometimes made against witches that they possessed teats in their anuses which were sucked by their familiars. Murray, *Witch-Cult in Western Europe*, pp. 95-6.

L

a derivative of the experience of satisfying the yearning of the bowels. Roheim has argued that the primitive medicine man, who shoots excrement symbols into his patients, similarly reverses the acts of his mother.[1]

24. *Urethral impulses.*

Less studied but no less important in their consequences than the needs of the bowels are those of the bladder. Just as the anticipation of the pleasure of eating or defecating turns the needs of the stomach into desires and appetites, so the memory of the pleasure of micturating, when combined with the need, forms the corresponding appetite. Any observer of children, even if he is without psycho-analytic training, must have noticed the extreme pleasure with which the little boy relieves his bladder. It is this pleasure which first draws his attention to those organs which are later destined to play so large a role, not only in his own life, but in that of the race. But the early valuation of the penis is also largely due, like the valuation of the faeces, to the transference of impulses from other spheres. There is no doubt that the penis, soon after it is first discovered, becomes another substitute for the nipple, and perhaps children of both sexes pass through a stage of conscious or unconscious fellatio fantasies on their road from infantile oral desires to adult sexual wishes. Probably at some stage desire, consciously or unconsciously, to suck the penis of another person ; but to attain the adult sexual impulse, the little girl has only to substitute her vagina for her mouth while the little boy must first project this impulse upon a woman before making a similar substitution.

[1] Roheim, *Nach dem Tode des Urvaters*, Imago, ix.

The analogy between the act of sucking and the act of coitus has not escaped some pre-psycho-analytic authors. Havelock Ellis writes that the 'erectile nipple corresponds to the erectile penis, the eager watery mouth of the infant to the moist and throbbing vagina, the vitally albuminous milk to the vitally albuminous semen.'[1] The same author has unearthed from Cleland's erotic novel, *The Memoirs of Fanny Hill*, a reference to 'the compressive exsuction with which the sensitive mechanism of that part (the vagina) thirstily draws and drains the nipple of love.'[2] The same analogy is probably at the basis of the common primitive belief that conception follows the eating of certain kinds of food. We should expect those kinds which are supposed to be especially potent to be phallic symbols. Such beliefs seem to be expressions of the fellatio fantasies which so often form the connecting link between early oral and urethral impulses and the later genital desires.

Just as the habit of stimulating the mouth or anus with the finger in the absence of a genuine oral or anal need may develop as a reassurance against a neurotic anxiety, so the habit of masturbation may arise for analogous reasons in the urethral stage. It is commonest in children who must enjoy micturation but who are compelled by their elders to restrict this pleasure. Masturbation is perhaps originally the reassurance which reproduces some of the senations of micturation and thereby guarantees their urethral potency.[3]

[1] *Studies in the Psychology of Sex*, 2nd ed., iii. 18.   [2] *Ib.* 19, n.
[3] Money-Kyrle, *The Meaning of Sacrifice*, 43-4.

25. *Genital impulses.*

The sexual need is terminated by an orgasm which is produced by the rhythmical stimulus of the sex organs, and one might suppose that some kind of masturbation would be learnt as the most appropriate removal. But we know that in practice a more complicated performance is generally preferred. The need, which is determined by the pressure of the various sexual fluids upon the walls of their containing glands, or by their action when discharged into the blood stream, evokes the seeking of a means, that is, a mate. The additional presence of the means evokes the act of penetration, and the stimulus of penetration sets off the final ejaculation.

We have argued in the last section that something very like the true genital impulse to penetrate, or to be penetrated by, the sexual organs of a member of the opposite sex can develop from pre-genital impulses alone. We may now suggest that if the reactions to these other impulses had not paved the way, some simpler procedure than that of coitus might be acquired to still the sexual need. The oral impulse necessitates an object; for we cannot eat without first seeking food. But anal and urethral impulses do not seek to incorporate something which they are without ; they excrete something which is superfluous. At first sight, the male sexual impulse would seem to belong to this latter category.

We have argued that infantile oral impulses survive their real utility because they remove false threats.[1]

[1] Chap. iv, 22.

The threat of hunger survives in the unconscious and compels a continual search for some mother symbol who shall for ever remove the possibility of need. This search may result, among other things, in fellatio fantasies in girls and in projected fellatio fantasies in boys. Finally, by substituting the vagina for the mouth, the act of coitus can remove symbolically a fictitious oral threat which has survived from infancy, as well as the real genital need. We may thus suggest that it is partly because of the fusion of the genital need with the pre-genital threat, that coitus, which requires an object, is usually preferred to masturbation.

This theory, however, is open to the objection that it does not easily apply to non-mammals, who cannot, like us, begin their sexual education at their mother's breasts. We must conclude, therefore, that ontogenesis cannot give an adequate explanation of the sexual impulse. If, as some Behaviourists seem to believe, the reactions of the organism were due solely to environment unassisted by heredity, oral, anal, and urethral impulses might have developed much as they do. But, at least among non-mammals, the reaction which secured the ejaculation of those fluids which excite the sexual impulse would have been simpler for the individual and useless to the race. Only inheritance can explain why an excretive impulse should require an object.[1]

[1] All needs might be qualified as either excretive or ingestive. The reaction appropriate to an excretive need is a final removal unpreceded by a seeking, but the correct response to an ingestive need includes the seeking of a means. The sexual need is an exception, for, although it is excretive, it demands an object.

3. Love.[1]

The peculiar emotions which accompany the genital impulse are not made up solely of those personal bodily sensations which the preparation for, and execution of, the act of coitus would seem to require. For beyond these personal sensations there is a sense of unity with another person. This sense of unity has seemed to many too ethereal to be reduced to simpler feelings, and therefore something non-animal within us, the proof of an origin which is partly divine. In fact the poetical philosopher is apt to pounce on just such feelings of unity and sympathy and to regard them as his last refuge from the ravages of science. But science, which is a spiritual descendent of Prometheus, is impudent, and has ever refused to be shown its place. Soon it will violate the secret recesses of the soul. The first attack may not be successful, but it will be repeated, with relentless persistence, until the citadel is won.

According to associationist psychologists, sympathy is either the sensation of our own imitation of other people's gestures, or the recollection of what this sensation would be. This theory has been shown by the intuitionists to be inadequate.[2] But it has at least the merit that it requires no new fundamental postulates. Intuitionism, on the other hand, pre-supposes some kind of telepathic communication. And, though the theory of telepathy is no logical impossibility, there seems to be nothing in nature,

[1] *Cf.* Chap. iii, 2227.
[2] Scheler, *Wesen und Formen der Sympathie.*

except a lack of mechanical ingenuity in devising alternative -explanations of the facts, which could lead anyone to suppose that it was true. Therefore it is along associationist lines that we must first look for an account of the development of sympathy in general, and of the sense of unity between lovers in particular.

When we imagine that we intuitively perceive something in another, we are in all probability projecting something which was originally within ourselves, and this is true whether what we see is contemptible or sublime. If, when we disapprove of others, we are really seeing something which is in ourselves, it is no less true that we have created our purest gods in our own image. For this reason Goethe wrote ' *Du gleichst dem Geist den du begreifst.*' We therefore resemble the minds which we can understand, and cannot understand those which we do not resemble.

Now we resemble others when they imitate us as well as when we imitate them. According to the old associationist theory, we understand others because we imitate or have imitated them. But it would seem more correct to say that we understand others because they imitate us in something which we do, or have done, or would have liked to do. This distinction may seem pedantic, but it will be of service, for it corresponds with the difference between introjection and projection.

31. *Projection.*

A desire is the sensation of a need plus the idea of ourselves realizing the means to its removal. But sometimes the desire is disowned. The sensation of our need is there, but it is accompanied by the idea of someone else realizing the means. A desire may be disowned and attributed to someone else for two reasons, either because it is incompatible with other desires, or because it is incompatible with possibilities. Thus the repressed sadist sees cruelty in others, and the father who has failed to realize his ambitions will project them upon his sons.

It is probable that we are all bi-sexual, that we inherit dispositions to the sexual acts of members of the opposite sex as well as to those of our own, and that the pre-genital desires of our childhood might have developed indifferently into desires appropriate to either sex. In some individuals the homosexual (subject-homosexual) impulses are repressed and manifest themselves only as sublimations. But in so far as anyone completely represses these impulses he will be devoid of sympathy with his mistress and unable to understand or reflect her feelings. He will be incapable of that sense of unity which to many is the main value of the sexual experience. More often, however, the homosexual impulses are not completely repressed, but disowned, either because they are impossible or because they are incompatible with other impulses. Just as the disappointed father projects unrealized ambitions upon his sons, or the mother upon her daughters, so the disappointed masculinity of the girl may find a vicarious satisfaction in a manly lover, or the disappointed femininity of the boy in a womanly mistress.

The normal girl gives up her masculinity only because it is incompatible with her physical structure,not because she is ashamed of it. But the normal boy gives up his femininity not only because it is incompatible with his body but also because it is incompatible with his pride. Therefore he is more likely to repress it completely and to possess a defective capacity for sympathy with his mistress, than a woman is with her lover.

But what is only projected, and not utterly repressed, can still be vicariously enjoyed. The sense of unity between lovers in the sexual act, which is the limit of sympathy, seems to require as one of its conditions that the heterosexual impulses of each partner shall really correspond to the projected homosexual impulses of the other, so that each experiences vicariously what he or she has disowned.[1]

32. *Introjection.*

When others imitate us in something which we do, have done, or would have liked to do, we project our feelings upon them. And when we imitate others we introject their feelings. The old associationist theory attributed sympathy to an introjection or imitation. Perhaps the reason why it has seemed inadequate to so many acute introspectionists is because what is introjected, although it is derived from others, is thought

---

[1] Where this condition is not fulfilled, the love relationship is imperfect and unlikely to be permanent. Since its presence or absence can seldom be determined beforehand, a satisfying sexual partner is unlikely to be discovered without trial and error,

of as our own. But, in sympathy, we do not merely reciprocate the feelings of another ; we attribute them to him

Introjection, moreover, is not an ultimate process, but the re-introjection of something which has previously been projected. Indeed, we must first learn to desire, that is, to associate a sensation of a need with an image of ourselves attaining the means to its removal, before we can project desires upon others, that is, associate the sensation (or idea) of someone else attaining a means with an idea (or sensation) of the corresponding need. In sympathy we disown a desire and project it upon someone else. But once we have learnt to sympathize with others we can appropriate or introject their desires, though in doing so we are really only retaking our own possessions. The projected desire (*i.e.*, the sensation or idea of a need plus the sensation or idea of someone else realizing the means) may re-excite the original desire (*i.e.*, the idea of us attaining it ourselves). That is, we may introject or reintroject an old desire. It is this process of introjection that the associationists used to offer as an account of sympathy when they said that sympathy is the sensation of our own imitation of other people's gestures, or of the recollection of what these sensations would be. But, in fact this process does not give sympathy, in the sense that sympathy is the attribution to others of our own desires, but identification, which is the attribution to ourselves of other people's desires, even though they were once our own.

The pre-genital part of the total sexual impulse is

not immediately directed to the sex organs and may be common to both sexes. Such impulses are infectious when they occur in one partner and correspond to dispositions in the other, and, in general, the desires of each are increased by the mutual introjection of complementary impulses. The female monkey who presents her buttocks in imitation of her sire,[1] admirably illustrates this process. In like manner among human beings the excitement of the preliminary pre-genital activities, such as kissing and embracing, are transferred. It is this mutual infection of emotion which seems to constitute the chief element in that sense of the expansion of the ego which accompanies the act of love.

33. The sense of unity.

The sense of unity between lovers is not sympathy alone nor identification alone, but a mixture of the two. At the risk of over-simplification we may say that it is due partly to the projection and vicarious enjoyment of disowned homosexual desires[2] and partly to the introjection of desires which are pre-genital.

Many would no doubt object that the sense of unity is debased by a sexual derivation, and would support their disagreement by the argument that it is strongest between those who have no sexual relations with

[1] Cf. Chap. i, 227.

[2] ' Moi je doublais mon bonheur par celui que je lui donnais ; car j'ai toujours eu la faiblesse de composer les quatres cinquièmes de mes jouissances de la somme de celles que je procurais à l'être charmant qui me les fournissait.' Casanova, Garnier's ed. i, 322.

each other. But among normal couples this feeling of unity may be observed to follow a periodic curve. Its intensity increases with desire and reaches a maximum during the sexual act. After complete satiation the intensity again falls rapidly until the partners, who so recently felt themselves to be one person both physically and mentally, are again two separate individuals with independent interests. Among lovers whose conscious sexual impulses are inhibited the feeling may be more permanent, but it is certainly less strong.

4. *The distortion of impulses.*

The same situation is sometimes both a threat and a means, so that, if the threat predominates, the seeking is inhibited. Often an equally satisfactory means is discovered by trial and error and the inhibited seeking is abandoned. But sometimes, no alternative is found to the removal of the need, so that the inhibition remains insecure. The impulse which would evoke a precariously inhibited seeking of this nature may remain conscious, when it is said to be *suppressed*, or it may apparently completely disappear, when it is said to be *repressed*.

Whether or not an impulse corresponding to a seeking is suppressed or repressed probably depends upon the neural level of the inhibition. Consciousness seems to be the correlate of certain central neural processes in the cerebral cortex or the sensorium. Thus we may suppose that, if a nervous process is inhibited after it reaches this level, the corresponding impulse remains conscious, and only its translation into action is suppressed, but that, if it is inhibited before it reaches this level, the corresponding impulse is repressed.

It is worth while at this point to raise the question whether a repressed impulse is simply non-existent or whether it exists in an unconscious state. Since nervous activity in the cortex is known to be accompanied by mental states, it is natural to suppose that all nervous activity may also be accompanied by mental events even if they are dissociated from the main body of consciousness and so beyond the range of introspection. If, therefore, we may make this assumption, mental impulses corresponding to persistent seekings, inhibited before the central level, must also exist as desires dissociated from the main body of consciousness.

A large part of psycho-analytical theory may perhaps be most easily made plausible if the same argument is extended and we assume not only two consciousnesses, but a whole hierarchy corresponding to different levels of the nervous system. This hypothesis will enable us to visualize how an infantile impulse may undergo a whole series of distortions, each of which is successively unravelled by analysis in the reverse order to that in which it originally developed.

Certain psycho-analysts, especially those with anthropological leanings, maintain that repressions developed in our forefathers by the conditions of their culture are inherited by us. Roheim, for instance, attributes much of present-day repression to the reactions of primeval man to the murder of his father.

But this presupposes the unlikely hypothesis of the inheritance of acquired characters. It seems more probable that, if repressions are inherited at all, they were not derived from previous learned adaptations to a social environment, but from a succession of spontaneous modifications, which most closely anticipated what had to be learnt. Intelligence often anticipates evolution, for both produce what is of survival value. This may give the erroneous impression that the products of intelligence are inherited.

It is at least certain that a great part of repression is due to early environment, rather than to the inheritance of innate or acquired inhibitions. The oral, anal, and urethral impulses of the child are successively repressed. And, if nothing prevents the discovery of satisfactory means to genital needs, they are largely abandoned ; for the needs themselves have changed and the old means no longer satisfy them. To some extent, however, these old pre-genital impulses survive unconsciously, whether or not they remain appropriate, have lost their appropriateness, or never were appropriate. Of this remnant, some reappear as preliminaries (such preliminaries may be called ' normal perversions ') to the adult sexual act, and others as those useful desexualized activities which are known as sublimations.

If, however, the genital impulses are themselves repressed by the Œdipus complex at the beginning of their development, the pre-genital desires also remain unsatisfied. Sublimations alone are an insufficient outlet, and, since they cannot appear as appendages of the normal sexual impulse, they can find an outlet only in perversions or neurotic symptoms.

A perversion is a very slightly distorted edition of the original pre-genital impulse. It occurs when the pre-genital repression breaks down. A symptom, on the other hand, is a highly distorted substitute for the original. In this it resembles the sublimation, but, unlike the sublimation, it is wholly involuntary and gives no pleasure to the ego. It occurs when the pre-genital repression is maintained.

Thus, if genital impulses are not repressed, pre-genital desires remain only mildly active and are satisfied partly in genital preliminaries and partly in sublimations. If genital impulses are repressed, the pre-genital desires remain strongly active, and give rise either to a neurosis or a perversion, to a neurosis if the pre-genital repression is also strong, and to a perversion if it is weak.

Although the main source of sublimations, perversions, and neuroses is to be found in pre-genital impulses, genital tendencies may also find distorted expression, and this may be again either a sublimation valued by the ego and by society, a perversion enjoyed by the one but detested by the other, or a neurosis deplored by both.

All psychological classifications are to some extent arbitrary, but they are often convenient, and when their limitations are not forgotten they do not mislead. We may therefore classify perversions, sublimations, and neuroses according to the type of unconscious impulse which is mainly concerned in their formation. The best known and most investigated of these are the oral, anal, and urethral tendencies, each of which is responsible for certain common groups of derivatives which we may consider in turn.

41. *Perversions.*

It is difficult to isolate perversions which are purely oral, but the following list is composed of activities which have an important oral component. Kissing would not usually be classed as a perverse activity, but, since it has retained its manifest erotic element and is pre-genital, it corresponds to our definition. It does not occur among many peoples,[1] and it may therefore be classed as a perversion especially common to Europeans. Among less approved oral perversions may be mentioned drug-taking, which has often a conscious erotic charm, cannibalism, necrophagy, and coprophagia, which are complicated by anal elements, and fellatio and cunnilinctus, which are fused with urethral and genital impulses.

In the list of anal perversions coprophagia occurs again, although it has a partly oral origin. Flagellation is mainly an anal erotic interest, but it also has oral elements, while pederasty is partly genital. For certain individuals the act of defecation is an almost complete substitute for any other sexual activity.

The list of urethral perversions is not so long, possibly because the subject has received less attention, but urolagnia, which comprises the perversions of urinating

[1] Malinowski, *Sexual Life of Savages*, 278-9.

over someone, or of being urinated upon, or of drinking urine, appears to be not uncommon.[1]

All these perversions are substitutes for the normal sexual act which has become repressed. In so far as they do not remove the real needs of sex they are inadequate removals or seekings. But they may give a partial satisfaction to pre-genital impulses.

42. *Sublimations.*

Whereas perversions are always the almost undisguised expressions of pre-genital tendencies, sublimations and neurotic symptoms are much more distorted and difficult to trace to their origin. Sublimations and symptoms, moreover, may be reaction formations against pre-genital impulses, as well as disguised expressions of them. They may therefore be composed of avoidances as well as of seekings. The latter type we may call positive, the former negative.

Good examples of positive and negative oral sublimations are smoking and vegetarianism, and of anal sublimations, productivity and thrift. Ambition is supposed to be derived from urethral impulses, but, although the connection has been empirically well founded, I do not think it has been adequately explained. The fear of damp, and the almost obsessional airing of sheets, which is a special characteristic of the English housewife, is probably as much a negative urethral sublimation as a rational reaction to our climate.

[1] Havelock Ellis, *Studies in the Psychology of Sex*, 1929, Chap. ii.

M

43. *Neuroses.*

In neurotic symptoms, positive and negative reactions are generally fused into a unity which is hard to separate. The psychotic withdrawal of all interest from the external world is a typical regression to the oral level of the infant, and the refusal to take nourishment, which is so common in melancholia, must be an oral reaction. The obsessional neuroses provide many illustrations of the fusion of anal impulses with their corresponding reaction formations. Many cases have been reported in the psycho-analytic journals, but they are too complicated to be summarized with ease.[1]

44. *Re-education.*

The perversions are inadequate substitutes for sexual reactions, but to some extent they satisfy pre-genital needs. Often, however, these needs are not real but only false threats. The sublimations are also inadequate or irrelevant reactions to the situations which first called them forth. They seek means which inadequately resemble the means to the removal of the organic need, or they avoid situations which irrelevantly resemble real threats. But they generally acquire a secondary relevance or adequacy which makes them really useful, even though they do not derive their energy from this rational source.

The neuroses, however, are not only inadequate or irrelevant substitutes for some other reaction, but they have no secondary adequacy or relevance. They are not only entirely useless, but, in so far as they

[1] One or two further examples are given in Chap. vi, 1.

interfere with other impulses, they are extremely painful. It is against such symptoms especially that the process of re-education known as psycho-analysis is most effective.

In analysis, the essential process is the making conscious of repressions. Many of these are then seen to have lost their relevance or never to have possessed a relevance. The seekings which are indispensable to the removal of real needs are freed. The symptoms thus become unnecessary and generally disappear; or, if they do not do so, they are also analysed and their inadequacy or irrelevance exposed. The process of psycho-analysis is, however, long and difficult; for the inhibitions which it must uncover before it can succeed are those of early infancy. It is therefore futile to recommend a patient to overcome his scruples and lead a normal sexual life, for this is the one thing which, until he is analysed, he cannot do.

CHAPTER VI

THE EFFECTS AND VALUE OF PSYCHOLOGY

So far, we have been concerned with the nature and general structure of psychology, and with the psychological history of the race, of culture, and of the individual. In this last chapter we shall inquire about the effects and value of this science.

In attempting to estimate the value of psychology we are confronted at the outset by special difficulties which do not impede the investigation of the value of any other science. We find that most other sciences assist the realization of certain common desires, and, when we have described how this service is performed, we feel that our duty has been accomplished and that we are not called upon to inquire further whether or not these desires are themselves justified. Thus we may say that physics is useful because it gives us electric light, or that medicine has value because it cures disease. We take it for granted that electric light and health are themselves desirable. But psychology, unlike other sciences, does not merely facilitate the realization of desires ; it alters them and causes some to be abandoned as irrational. Thus it is much more difficult to determine the value of psychology than of any other science. For this reason we shall first try to anticipate the probable effects of psychology before considering whether or not these effects will be welcome.

The organism, we have seen, is so constructed that it reacts to the primary stimuli of injuries and needs until they are removed ; that it reacts to the secondary stimuli of threats as if they were primary and so avoids real injuries and needs ; and that its removal and avoidance reactions often involve the seeking of means. We have seen further that irrelevant avoidances and inadequate seekings sometimes develop and that irrelevant avoidances may be superimposed on adequate seekings. Lastly, we have seen that this type of irrelevant avoidance, which might be called irrelevant inhibition, can be eliminated by psycho-analysis, and that the same process of re-education also destroys other inappropriate impulses. It seems likely that this science is destined to inaugurate an era of increasing self-knowledge in the world at large. Here we shall discuss its remote effects not only on the individual who is himself analysed but on the society and even the race which is brought up under its influence.

1. *Individual consequences.*

We have argued that not only neurotic symptoms and perversions, but also sublimations, are made up partly of irrelevant avoidances or inadequate seekings or both. We have now to inquire whether all or only some of these are likely to be eliminated by self-knowledge. But to do this we must first distinguish carefully between those irrelevant and inadequate reactions which possess a secondary real value and those which do not.

11. *Negative symptoms.*

Irrelevant avoidances which are symptoms make up what psycho-analysts call the reaction formations in the neuroses. Thus the phobias and the compulsions are characteristic neurotic avoidances. A phobia of snakes, for example, is an irrelevant avoidance of a particular phallic symbol. Such avoidances are superimposed upon seekings. It is not quite so obvious that the compulsions are irrelevant avoidances because they are rather more complicated. But although they may be fused with inadequate seekings, their foundation is a reaction formation, or an avoidance. Thus, in a case quoted by Freud, a young girl could not sleep without a lengthy ceremonial to prevent the possibility of her bolster touching the end of her bed. The contact between these objects symbolized to her the union of her parents which, in her ceremonial, she symbolically and irrelevantly prevented.[1]

[1] A case reported by Reik (*Endphasen des religiosen und des zwangsneurotischen Glaubens*, Imago xvi, 26) well illustrates the fusion of an adequate seeking with an irrelevant avoidance. A neurotic young woman suffered from the obsessional fear that she might have left the tap on in the bathroom and from the compulsion to go there several hundred times each day to make quite sure. The analysis recalled a scene with her bridegroom, in which she had feared that he might have an ejaculation. Her compulsive action, in which she had to turn the tap on in order to see that it was properly turned off, symbolized at once her desire to secure this event and her reaction against this desire.

Irrelevant avoidances of this nature have no secondary relevance and they tend to disappear when they are understood.

12. *Negative sublimations.*

Irrelevant avoidances that have a secondary relevance form one type of sublimation. Thus the statesman who devotes his life to the protection of his country against a remote danger, may owe his energy to a symbolic or irrelevant resemblance between the idea of foreign aggression and the unconscious fear of castration. But if the danger happens to be real, this type of anxious patriotism has a secondary relevance, and is a sublimation rather than a neurotic symptom.

Irrelevant avoidances of this kind, which have acquired a secondary relevance, may survive the exposure of their first motive.

13. *Positive symptoms.*

Inadequate removals and seekings without secondary adequacy make up the positive side of the neuroses. They may be best illustrated in hysterical symptoms. Thus a hysteric in situations in which the normal man would have an erection, may develop a deep blush, or a swelling of the foot, or react in some equally inadequate manner. Such reactions do not merely have no secondary adequacy, but they are usually acutely painful. They are inadequate not merely because the adequate reaction does not happen to have been discovered but because it is actively inhibited. To cause their disappearance it is not sufficient to disclose their inadequacy, which is usually obvious enough. It is also necessary to discover the irrelevance of the inhibition. Analysis can and does make both these discoveries and therefore tends to eliminate such symptoms.

14. *Positive sublimations.*

Inadequate seekings with a secondary adequacy make up what we may term the positive sublimations. Thus the statesman who devotes his energies to the conquest of another country may owe his motive to an unconscious desire to conquer a woman. But aggressive imperialism, if it is successful, may have a secondary adequacy as a reaction to a real economic need. If so, it may survive the disclosure of the inadequacy of its unconscious motive.

15. *Perversions.*

Lastly we may distinguish a type of removal or seeking which is semi-adequate, and I think that the perversions should be included in this class. A perversion is a regression to an earlier level of development. It may be adequate to infantile needs, but it is not wholly adequate to the adult needs into which these earlier ones have developed. Thus the sexual impulse is partly developed from, and includes, the oral, anal, and urethral needs of infancy. But if the genital reaction is inhibited, the sexual needs of the adult cannot be satisfied. The perversion, however, which is a regression to an earlier reaction that may have been adequate to the pre-genital needs of the infant, is still a partial satisfaction. Therefore, the perversion, unlike the neurotic symptom, does not leave the despondence of complete futility, and it is in consequence more difficult to cure. If the inhibitions of the genital response are understood, the perversion will be largely replaced by a more adequate response. But when it involves no serious inconvenience it may survive as a part of the preliminaries of the adequate genital reaction.

16. *The elimination of inadequate and irrelevant reactions.*

The fundamental effect of psycho-analysis is, as we have seen, the elimination of inadequate or irrelevant reactions. With the growth of self-knowledge, therefore, the neuroses, which are wholly inappropriate in this sense, will tend to disappear. The perversions, which are partly inadequate, will tend to be replaced by more adequate impulses ; while the sublimations, which possess a secondary adequacy or relevance (i.e. which are ego-syntonic), will be likely to survive the loss of the motives which originally produced them.

We may inquire whether, in a society of completely enlightened individuals, sublimations ever could arise. It would seem at first sight that if children discovered, or were taught, the real means to all their needs immediately these first occurred, and were never deceived by false threats, they might be deprived of those errors which would later be so useful. But it is inconceivable that such a condition could occur ; for children must teach themselves by trial and error, and they acquire the mistakes which develop into sublimations before they can understand enough to learn from others. False threats of castration in particular and of aphanisis in general, inhibit the discovery of adequate seekings so that a great variety of inadequate substitutes are quickly developed.

If, however, self-knowledge ever began to endanger the sublimations of the child, the adult, who had learnt their secondary value, would be likely to postpone such a destructive education.

2. *Social consequences.*

To the psycho-analyst, the great mass movements of society are collective neuroses or collective sublimations. We have seen that the effect of that deepening of self-knowledge which psychology will bring to the world will tend to eliminate neurosis in the individual. We have now to inquire which of the social manifestations have no secondary relevance or adequacy. These, since they are comparable to the negative and positive symptoms of the individual, seem doomed to ultimate extinction. The process may be slow, and it may not be continuous, but it will be sure. There may be dark ages in the future as in the past. But from time to time, there will be waves of enlightenment which will surpass all their predecessors, and there are no sands of irrationality which will not be eventually submerged.

We shall attempt here to separate the rational from the irrational in religion, morality, and politics, and therefore to predict their fate.

2. *Social consequences—religious.*

Religion is made up of avoidances as well as of seekings, and the negative side is almost certainly the older. Thus when Freud speaks of an obsessional neurosis as a private religion, he is thinking chiefly of the negative and more archaic side of religion, for the obsessional neurosis is composed chiefly of avoidances.

211. *Negative religion.*

Negative religion may be roughly sub-divided into two kinds, according to whether what is avoided is the threat of punishment for rebellion against God, or whether it is the impulse to rebellion itself.[1]

We know that, when the Œdipus complex is repressed, the hostile tendencies are often projected and inverted against the self and feared as a threat of punishment. It is this threat from the inverted hostile impulses of the self which is feared in the first type of negative religion. The religious melancholics who suffer from it are tortured by constant fear of hell-fire or of the wrath of God. Their attempt at propitiation by self-punishment provides some outlet for their inverted aggressiveness, and, where the sexual impulse is also inverted, the penance may give a masochistic satisfaction.

The first step in the understanding of a pathological fear of the wrath of God exposes this fear as an irrelevant avoidance of an inverted aggressive impulse. The next step exposes this inverted impulse as inadequate because it is directed against the self instead

[1] *Cf.* Chap. iv, 14.

of against the external object which originally provoked it. Thus at a certain phase in the process of enlightenment, the fear of God is replaced by a more primary hate of Him, which may alternate or co-exist with an even stronger love.

The second type of negative religion which we defined as the fear of rebelling against God, rather than as the fear of the wrath of God, occurs when the aggressive impulses are repressed without being inverted against the self. Just as the obsessional neurotic devotes his energies to the avoidance of any action which resembles, however remotely, the execution of his unconscious hostile wishes, so the negatively religious man of the second type is always over-anxious lest he should do anything hostile to his God. His religion is a mass of ceremonials and taboos. He must pray in a certain manner in order to prevent the intrusion of blasphemous thoughts. He must fast on certain occasions, like the savage whose totem is taboo, to repress his theophagic inclinations. And he must undertake no enterprise on the Sabbath lest he should repeat the dismemberment of his totem god which once occurred on this day. Analysis would convince him that his elaborate rites avoid the symbol rather than the reality of revolt and that they are therefore irrelevant. Thus he also would pass into a stage in which his irrelevant obsessional avoidances of revolt against God were replaced by a conscious ambivalence.

If such an individual's understanding of his own motives terminated with the realization that he hated

God, he would remain ambivalent, and might alternate between militant atheism and passionate belief. But the avoidance of revolt determined by the more powerful love would at least be relevantly directed against a conscious hostility rather than irrelevantly against mere symbols.

If, however, his self-understanding continued to deepen, he would soon realize that God was a symbol for his father, who would then become the object of his conscious ambivalence. In other words, he would realize that his hate of God was inadequate because it was directed against the wrong object. The last and final stage of the analysis would be to show that this hate is in itself inadequate.

There was nothing psychologically inadequate or irrelevant about the original construction of the Œdipus complex, except in so far as the incestuous impulses which started the whole process were partly founded not on real needs but on false threats of needs. But what is inadequate and irrelevant is the survival of hate long after the time at which it might have been really appropriate. The basis of the Œdipus complex of the adult, which is the persistence of incestuous impulses, is perhaps not even wholly inadequate. The persistent unconscious seeking of the mother seems to be made up of two parts, one adequate and one irrelevant. In so far as she is sought as a means to the removal of real oral and genital needs, she is sought adequately. But in so far as the motive for this seeking is loneliness, *i.e.*, a false threat of hunger and aphanisis, the seeking is an irrelevant avoidance of a false threat, *i.e.*, it is due to a neurotic anxiety. Therefore one element in the continued seeking of the mother who was known in the first months of infancy is not so much the seeking of an object which inadequately resembles a real means, as the seeking of an object that no longer exists. Analysis cannot prevent us from seeking the impossible. But, what is more important, it can convince us that our fathers are no longer the real impediments to our desires and that to hate them is to hate inadequately. Freud seems to believe that this hate is indestructible and a permanent danger to society,[1] but we may perhaps adopt the more optimistic view that it is preserved by an unconscious misunderstanding of the causes of frustration and that it can be analysed away.[2]

212. *Positive religion.*

Positive religion is not made up of avoidances but of seekings. The dominant note is not the fear of the wrath of God or fear of revolting against Him, but an intense desire for an ever more intimate union with Him. For the psycho-analyst it is not hard to understand the development of these impulses. The demands of the child are insatiable and doomed to disappointment. All his life he dimly remembers the mother of his first months who seemed to fulfil all his needs, and all his life he seeks her. She is the ideal woman whom he will some day meet and who will

[1] *Das Unbehagen in der Kultur.*
[2] For a continuation of this argument see R. Money-Kyrle, " A Psychologist's Utopia," *Psyche*, April, 1931.

make him happy, and unless he realizes that this dream is an impossibility, his marriages are likely to be numerous and of short duration.

Paradoxical as it may sound, one of the first mother-substitutes to which the child partially transfers his intense affection is his father. At this age he makes little distinction between the sexes, and, when his mother ceases to satisfy him completely, he readily expects what he misses from that other member of his family whom he sees more rarely and who, in consequence, has less opportunity to disappoint him.

The father is, therefore, not only the main impediment to the realization of the incestuous impulses but also the object to which they are first most likely to be transferred. As the impediment to the realization of the incestuous impulse towards the mother, the father becomes an object of hate. But the love which is transferred to him represses this hate. In the inverted Œdipus complex, even the rest of the love which is not transferred to the father is projected upon him and inverted to the self, so that the child not only loves his father as he loved his mother, but desires to be loved by him.

Just as the mother disappoints the first incestuous desires, so too the father disappoints them in their inverted form. But the child, once he has formed this concept, never forgets it and seeks it in his idea of God.[1]

We have next to inquire how far the seeking of God in positive religion is inadequate, and to what extent it is likely to survive the spread of a knowledge of psychology.

[1] Flügel, *The Psycho-Analytic Study of the Family*, chap. xiii.

If a personal God in the form of an all-loving and all-powerful father really existed he would undoubtedly satisfy some of the deepest yearnings of present humanity. He would be an adequate substitute for almost every human loss, and the certainty that this was so would remove almost every human fear. He would thus comfort the afflicted and calm the anxious. Unfortunately, however, the belief that such a being exists does not appear to be empirical, but seems to be founded upon desire alone. Thus we must conclude that positive religion can fulfil no real needs.

But how, then, are we to account for the fact that religion has comforted and still does comfort millions of individuals who without it would find life not only empty but intolerable ? We have seen that, although inadequate seekings cannot fulfil real needs, they may nevertheless remove false threats. Religion, therefore, since it combines an apparent adequacy with a real inadequacy, is perhaps of this nature, and is a relief only to neurotic anxiety.

The adult requires different means to satisfy his needs from those of the child, yet the absence of means which were necessary to the child may still operate as false threats. The absence of the mother was once a threat of hunger and pre-genital deprivation. The absence of the father was once a threat of his death, for which the child's unconscious had so often longed. The belief in the existence of the God who is a symbol of the mother and the father in one person removes the old threat of the loss of the mother and, at the same time, reassures the unconscious that it is no murderer.

Certain individuals cannot tolerate the loss of either of these supports. If they were to lose the ideal of God as the perfect mother their anxiety would be insupportable ; if they were to lose the ideal of God as the father, they would introject Him, and their unconscious hate would invert against themselves. Thus the idea of God is required as an object both of love and of hate. But this anxious love and this hate are both largely inappropriate impulses ; for the mother is no longer necessary[1] and the father is no longer an impediment to a vital desire. The completely normal individual in the course of his development would, I think, learn the irrelevance of some of his infantile anxieties, seek his real needs no longer in his mother but in some object more adequate to them in their adult form, would be reconciled with his father and introject him as a conscious part of his ego without danger. Such an individual would have few false threats which could only be removed by some fictitious means. The real deprivations and anxieties of this life would thus become not too heavy for him to bear, and he could dispense with his belief in God if the absence of evidence in His existence convinced him of the rationality of agnosticism.

Therefore, I think that the great edifice of religion, both in its positive and in its negative form, is doomed to fall before the slow but inevitable widening of self-consciousness which modern psychology will bring. Religion may be an exquisite illusion, but it is built on superfluous fears and hates. It thus involves

[1] *i.e.* the fear of being without her is due to a false threat.

N

anxiety, which is unnecessary for its devotees, and intolerance, which is tiresome for their opponents. We may regret the passing of much that was beautiful in the childhood of our culture, but we shall admit that the gain is greater than the loss.

22. *Social consequences—moral.*

Morality is supposed to consist of both precepts and prohibitions. The prohibitions are not only older but also more fundamental, for precepts, when analysed, are seen to be only the converse of prohibitions. Thus the taboo ' n'insulte pas tes parents de peur de mourir (aussitôt) ' is, as Reinach has pointed out, the origin of the precept ' honore tes parents afin que tu vives longtemps.'

Even the man who devotes his life to some great altruistic cause would probably admit, if he were honest, that his motives were partly the fear of the reproaches of his conscience if he failed to pull his weight in some way in society. And, in so far as his motives are not negative, but are due solely to altruistic love of his fellows, they are not the result of precepts and are therefore not moral. This is of course ultimately a matter of definition, but it would seem best in the interests of clarity to agree that morals are made up of prohibitions, and that purely positive impulses, in so far as they are not merely the converse of prohibitions, are not moral, however altruistic they may be.

We may therefore apply Reinach's definition of religion to morality and define it as ' un ensemble de

¹ Reinach, *Cultes, Mythes and Religions*, 1905, i, 5-6.

scruples qui font obstacle au libre exercice de nos facultés.'[1] Morality is thus akin to negative religion. In negative religion, a jealous God is believed to avenge all transgressions against His commands. In morals, this God is replaced by the conscience, or, to give it its modern and more comprehensive name, by the super-ego.[2] Formerly, morals were inseparable from negative religion ; the conscience was the voice of God. But the agnostic who refuses to accept the objective existence of God still has a conscience which is really the disembodied voice of God. Thus morality is a modern form of negative religion.

But whereas God is recognized by analysts as a projection of the father, the super-ego is supposed to be an introjection of him. There is, however, a great difference between introjecting the father into the ego and introjecting him as a super-ego ; the former strengthens the personality while the latter weakens it. The super-ego is distinct from the ego, and it differs from God only in that it is a disembodied edition of Him. Probably because the super-ego is not objectified but disembodied, it is regarded not as a projection but as an introjection. Since, however, it is distinct from the ego, it is still in a sense a projection.

The super-ego, or the Imago, is therefore a sort of disembodied God, a loved and needed object. But, paradoxically enough, the reason why it cannot be given up seems to be that it is hated as well as loved. If a loved object is lost it can be given up only if it is introjected. But to introject a loved object that is

[1] *Orpheus*, 4.   [2] *Cf*. Chap. iv, 16.

also hated is dangerous, for it involves the inversion of aggressive impulses that threaten to destroy the ego. The melancholic who does succeed in introjecting such an object is likely to terminate his life by suicide.

221. *The function of the Imago.*

We may now proceed to study the Imago in action. In the unconscious, the old incestuous impulses of childhood still from time to time strive towards their old object. Then they awaken the old sexual rivalry and aggressiveness which is perhaps an innate accompaniment of the sexual impulse. This aggressiveness or hate is directed first towards the Imago who is the symbol of the father who once suppressed them. But the Imago is also loved, so that the hate is repressed, projected, and inverted against the self, and felt as guilt. This lasts until the unconscious incestuous impulses are also inverted, and the whole cycle may end in some form of masochistic penance.

In negative religion this penance is more or less recognized for what it is, but in the unconscious and automatic morality, which has so largely replaced religion, it may be some form of neurotic suffering, or some misfortune which the subject does not even recognize as self-inflicted. Thus the case of a stockbroker has been recorded who periodically suffered heavy financial losses owing to temporary misjudgements which were really the result of his own inverted hate.

The same process of repression and inversion may follow, not only the periodic return of direct substitutes for the old incestuous impulses, but also their remotest sublimations. The inhibited impulses seek ever more inadequate substitutes for their original means, and each in turn may be followed by the same process of repression and inversion. Where the substitutes are still antisocial the Imago has thus been a far more efficient guardian of society than the law. But where they are no longer antisocial, and have secondary real value, both to the individual and society, the function of the Imago has been to produce useless and crippling neuroses.

222. *The analysis of the Imago.*

Having formed some idea of the inhibitions of the Imago, we have now to inquire how far these are irrelevant and therefore unlikely to survive. And, if they are mainly psychologically irrelevant, whether the society of the future is likely to relapse into the destructive anarchy characteristic of the family life of primeval man.

We may suppose that society will pass through the same stages of enlightment as the individual in analysis. The first stage will expose the irrelevant similarity between the inhibited sublimations and the incestuous impulses they symbolize. With this insight the neurotic inhibition of sublimations will decrease.

Many of the more direct sexual substitutes will be next freed. The impotent will become potent, the frigid more sensual, and the prude less chaste. But, at first, since the freed sexual impulses will still be only partially adequate substitutes for the original incestuous impulses, they will be unlikely to bring complete satisfaction. Discontented monogamists may become insatiably promiscuous in pursuit of an impossible goal.

Still further enlightenment will begin to disclose the partial inadequacy of the incestuous impulses themselves, for they unconsciously outlive the period in which they can really remove needs. They will also be shown to be irrelevant in so far as the threats which they seemed to remove were always false or have subsequently become so.[1] With this insight, the sexual activities, which have been already freed from inhibitions, will become simpler and more satisfying, and, although there may be less chastity than before, there will also be less useless promiscuity.

When the individualist of the future has realized the partial inadequacy and irrelevance of his unconscious incestuous impulses, and recognized his conscience as a derivative of his father, he will be less ambivalent towards it. It will frustrate him less; therefore it will not so easily excite his hatred. Some of the love, which was originally transferred to it from his mother, will find a more adequate substitute in a real woman; therefore he will feel less need to bask in the sunshine of its approval. Since it will be no longer hated it can be introjected without danger to the ego. Since it will be less loved it can be more easily given up as an object. Thus introjection into the ego will probably be its fate. The ego will be strengthened at the expense of the super-ego.

[1] I again allude to that part of the child's dependence upon its mother which is due to false threats of hunger, castration, and aphanisis.

With the final introjection of the Imago, not as a super-ego, but as a part of the ego, the individualist of the future will become the arbiter of his own morality.[1] Such a morality can be consciously modified ; but the basis of it will still be the standard of his Imago, that is, of his father and the series of father substitutes under whose influence he spent his early years. He will no longer be oppressed by this image ; he will become like it. The normal man does in fact, without analysis, approximate to this position.[2] But, in the past, those who have come up to this standard of normality have been few and far between, whereas, in the future, the moral individualist may be the rule.

Will the result be anarchy and the destruction of society ?[3] The basis of an individualist morality (*i.e.*, an ego morality as opposed to a super-ego morality) is transitive ; it is inherited, not as an innate possession, but as a form of property. Its survival in the future depends upon the present. It requires the continuity of family tradition. Thus, there is no reason why conscious morality should not survive the most complete enlightenment. But will this be a sufficient safeguard for society ? Although the unconscious and automatic basis of present morality will be largely lost, it will be less necessary. For the same process

---

[1] This process is never complete in actual analyses. Some part of the Imago is first projected upon the analyst and then, after the positive and negative transference has been analysed, it is reabsorbed into the ego.

[2] *Cf.* Money-Kyrle, *The Meaning of Sacrifice*, 55.

[3] *Cf.* Chap. iv, Introductory Remarks.

which proves it to be irrelevant discloses at the same time the psychological inadequacy of most of the anti-social impulses it was its function to repress.

It is unconscious hate bred of the real or imagined deprivations of humanity which is the real danger to society. These deprivations are partly self-inflicted and partly inflicted by society. That is, they result partly from our own irrelevant inhibitions and partly from the projected inhibitions of others. They are also partly not real deprivations at all, but false threats of these, which have survived from infancy. With an increase in self-knowledge, all these sources of real or imagined frustration will tend to dry up. There should be less unconscious hate, and less conscious discontent.

23. Social consequences—political.

Just as morals have become the modern equivalent of negative religion, so political idealism seems destined to fill the place in men's lives once occupied by positive religion. In positive religion, the perfect parents and the perfect home, which we dimly remember from our first infancy, are sought in a world of illusion beyond the grave. In political idealism, we seek to create the perfect government and the perfect state in this world, or to become ourselves the perfect race.

In political idealism, if we are not deluded, we do not ourselves expect to enjoy the utopia of our dreams. We do not, however, renounce them altogether but project them upon future generations. Political idealism is, therefore, more altruistic than religion.

But both are founded on the same unrenouncible desires, and both in consequence are almost equally unable to entertain the thought of the non-existence or impossibility of their ideals. Just as the religious man wilfully ignores the absence of all evidence for the existence of what he so much desires, so the political idealist will generally refuse to see the difficulties in the way of the realization of his utopia. Both also display the same intolerance and the same aggressiveness against those who differ from their views. Political idealism, however, seems to be somewhat nearer to reality than religion. It is not quite so irresponsibly certain of its results. It at least makes a pretence of testing the feasibility of the measures it proposes. And this tendency to scientific doubt and self-criticism seems to be increasing. Therefore political idealism may perhaps yet learn to test not only the feasibility but also the desirability of the new world before it has destroyed the old.

There is no subject which is more difficult to discuss impartially than politics, and even the psychologist may find his habitual impartiality desert him. He must first separate the problem of the realizability from that of the desirability of a given political ideal. The former problem belongs to economics, the latter to psychology. But it is easy to confuse the issue and to condemn as impossible an ideal which one dislikes. In this section, it is the psychological problem of the desirability of political ideals which will occupy us— though it will be difficult to resist the temptation to deviate occasionally into economics.

What a man desires for his class, his country, or his race, is a projection of what he desires for himself. If he could himself realize this desire he would not be so likely to project it. If he has repressed it severely, he may project it upon others without himself wishing it for them.[1] But if it is less severely repressed, or if it is not repressed at all, but merely under present conditions impossible, he is likely not only to project it upon others but also to desire it for them. In this way, a man transfers his ambitions to his children or builds ideals of what he wants society to become or avoid, and, if his capacity for altruistic projection is great, work towards such distant aims may become the main pre-occupation of his life.

But if a man is mistaken in what he thinks he wants or fears for himself, he is also likely to be mistaken in what he thinks he wants or fears for that projection of himself which is the world at large. Psychology, we have seen, helps the individual to discover what he really wants and what he need not avoid. Inadequate and irrelevant political ideals do no great harm to the individual who holds them, but they may be disastrous to his contemporaries and his successors. Therefore a psychology capable of eliminating such mistakes has a value to society at large.

Different objects may be equally adequate means to the same need, so that if the same situation evokes different desires in different people it does not necessarily follow that one desire must be less rational than

---

[1] E.g. he may project his sadism upon others and then join a society for the prevention of cruelty.

the other. Similarly, two political ideals may differ without either being necessarily mistaken. Therefore, we must not expect of psychology that it will eliminate all political conflict, but only that by exposing the irrelevance of many political ideals it will greatly diminish it.

Prynce Hopkins has pointed out that a man's politics are mainly determined by his Œdipus complex.[1] Perhaps it would be more correct to say that they are determined partly by this complex and partly by his social position. A man may have either a positive or a negative Œdipus complex, and he may have either a high or a low social position. The combinations of these two sets of factors give four typical kinds of politics, two reactionary and two progressive.

Those who have positive Œdipus complexes, if they are plutocrats, tend to identify the masses with their fathers and become reactionary, but if they are proletarians they tend to identify the rich with their fathers and as automatically become progressive. Of those who have negative Œdipus complexes the accident of social status has the opposite effect. If they are plutocrats they tend to identify the masses with the father, to whom they wish to surrender, and become masochistic revolutionaries, and if they are proletarians who see an image of their fathers in the rich, they may become masochistic reactionaries. Although there are numerous individual exceptions, this scheme seems to be a fairly general rule. Often the Œdipodean reaction is disowned and projected upon others, so that a

[1] Prynce Hopkins, *Fathers or Sons.*

politician may deceive himself, and his constituents, into the belief that he is disinterested, when he has merely projected the conscious part of his indignation upon the class with which he identifies himself.

Thus the politics of the majority of people, who feel strongly about such things, are probably expressions of projections of their own particular brand of Œdipus complex. Since the desires of this complex in the adult are largely inadequate or irrelevant, his political ideals, in so far as they have no secondary value, are also largely inadequate or irrelevant. They are therefore likely to be demotivated when he acquires a completer knowledge of himself.

Must we therefore conclude that a spread of knowledge of psychology will destroy all political ideals, and leave humanity profoundly apathetic about its future ? No, for there are individual desires which are adequate and rational, and among these there are many which we cannot ourselves fulfil and which it is easier to project upon others than utterly to renounce. Some of our ambitions may be inadequate, some of our sorrows and our fears may be irrelevant, but, when all this is allowed for, there must be many things which the most enlightened among us would still want and which we cannot have. A higher standard of comfort, more opportunity to choose our own work, greater physical strength and beauty and intellectual power— these are things which we may legitimately desire for our descendants if we cannot obtain them for ourselves. But less conscious and less rational motives are apt to lurk behind even these altruistic aspirations.

231. *Comfort.*

It is difficult to fix the standard of comfort which we really require, but it is certainly much more modest than we imagine that we want. For, as soon as our physical needs for nourishment and warmth have been satisfied, we demand of our homes that they shall require no drudgery to run, that they shall provide us privacy when we wish to be alone, and space for entertaining when we wish to see our friends. We next desire that they shall satisfy our private conceptions of elegance and beauty. And, if all these demands are satisfied we often wish them to be a medium of self-display. This last requirement can never be satisfied for everyone, for its fulfilment necessitates inequality. But it is also an irrelevant requirement, a reaction against a neurotic inferiority, which the spread of self-consciousness will in time remove.

At present, however, this demand for luxury as a means of self-display is very strong, and, in striving for it, our present culture is in danger of losing its far more rational requirements. There are two forms of this desire : the wish to display more luxury than others, and the wish to prevent others from displaying more luxury than oneself. Both appear to be reactions to a neurotic inferiority. But, whereas the first has a secondary value as an economic motive, the second has no compensating use. Both are apt to lurk behind the rational and quite different desire to be more comfortable oneself. And both appear in projected and altruistic forms. The conscious envy is repressed ; but it still seeks satisfaction behind the more rational desire to better our own position, or that of others with whom we identify ourselves.

It is especially important to distinguish the desire to be more comfortable ourselves from the desire to prevent others from becoming, or remaining, more comfortable than we are. For the economic methods of realizing these different political ideals are at present entirely different. A system of taxation designed to reduce inequality reduces at the same time the total wage-fund. And any political encouragement of capital which increases wages also increases inequalities. Thus the poor should realize that if they desire equality with the rich, they are likely to become themselves poorer in the process, and that, if they wish to raise their standard, they must permit the rich to become still richer.

It is, of course, possible that economists may eventually discover a method of realizing both these aspirations. But, since the ideal of equality is founded upon the irrational impulse of envy, in its direct or inverted form, it is doubtful whether the attempt would be worth the risk involved. Democracy is now, as often in the past, in the position of Æsop's dog. Perhaps, this time, it will learn from psychology that the other dog's bone is a reflexion, before it has lost its own.

232. *Work.*

More important than a high level of comfort is the power to do what we like with our time. Many people who have to work incessantly for their living imagine a state of idleness as a condition of extreme bliss. A short experience of this ideal would, however, soon convince them of their mistake, and teach them that what they really wanted was the power to choose their occupation rather than to have no occupation at all. It should not be beyond the capacity of economics to secure this more modest aim.

Just as a desire to restrict the comfort of others may be confused with the desire to increase our own, so may the wish to impede the freedom of other people take the place of the more rational wish to be the masters of our own time. In the name of freedom a gospel of state socialism is often preached which would regulate the smallest details of our lives. Under such a system a single father state would replace a multitude of capitalist employers. Those who now suffer under an economic slavery would find that socialism, as it is at present understood, although it might deprive others of their independence, would do nothing to increase their own. Psychology, by distinguishing these two motives, may do something to prevent experiments before their results can be clearly foreseen.

232. *Eugenics.*

The projected desire for physical and mental progress is rarer than the projected desire for comfort or freedom. But it is the fundamental motive of eugenists, and this type of political idealism is likely to become more common.

There are three stages in the development of the eugenic ideal. Firstly, there is the desire to rediscover as objects of love those perfect beings which we knew in our first infancy. This desire gives rise to the fantasies of romance and the longings of positive religion. Next, there is the tendency to give up this ideal as an object and to attempt to introject it. In this stage, we wish to be our ideals rather than to find them. The third and last stage involves the partial renunciation, as impracticable, of this desire for personal perfection and its projection upon our descendants, with whom we identify ourselves. Those who reach this stage are likely to become eugenists and active propagandists for racial improvement.

The ideal parents, which we all unconsciously still seek, would satisfy us if they could be found. Therefore, that part of the desire for them which is based on real needs rather than false threats, is rational, even if it cannot be fulfilled. The eugenic ideal is further removed from the original desire than its more direct expression in positive religion, but it is at least more likely to be fulfilled.

3. *Biological consequences.*

In the last two sections we have considered some of the individual and social consequences of an increase in self-knowledge. In this we shall attempt to foresee what effect, if any, this knowledge could have on evolution.

We have already raised the problem of whether psychology could endanger the sublimations of the individual. We may now enquire whether it could weaken the instincts of the race.

The neural structure which determines an instinct was selected, not because it led to the removal or avoidance of needs and injuries, but because it led to the survival of the offspring of the individuals who possessed it. No doubt what is best for survival is also often the shortest method of removing and avoiding needs and injuries. But this is not necessarily so. The neural structure we inherit thus predisposes us to remove our needs by a method which is of survival value to our children, but this method need not be the shortest path to the removal of these needs. If not, can instincts be unlearned, and replaced by reactions which are more satisfying to the individual but disastrous to the race ?[1]

[1] The most economical route from a given stimulus S_1 to the reaction Rf which finally removes it is the route in which $\leq$ Isn is a minimum, where the series Is_1 Is_2 . . . Isn . . . stands for the intensities of the series of stimuli S_1, S_2 . . . Sn . . . which successively occur during the series of reactions R_1, R_2 . . . Rn . . . Rf. I have assumed throughout this book as a fundamental principle that the individual must necessarily select the most economical route *that he has discovered.* In so far as we can identify pain with intensity of stimulus, this principle might be called the principle of negative hedonism. Observation, however, suggests that the human individual, at least, sometimes deliberately delays a final removal to some needs (*e.g.* nutritional, anal, urethral, sexual) in order to prolong and increase *pleasure.* What are we to make of this tendency ? Can it be reduced to a special form of negative hedonism ? Or must we postulate a ' positive hedonism ' by which the individual seeks certain kinds of stimuli, not merely as means to the removal of more primary stimuli, but also on their own account ? I cannot imagine what physiological principle can be correlated with such a positive hedonistic tendency. But, if it existed, it would doubtless protect instincts against the possibly destructive effects of the negative hedonism

o

I will take two examples. The sexual need is determined fundamentally by the periodic accumulation of certain chemical substances. When these are excreted the sexual need is temporarily at an end. It is however clear that the excretion of these substances by masturbation does not usually satisfy in the same way as the more complicated method which our instincts prescribe. Why not? Because masturbation does not satisfy our desire for an intimate union with some person whom we love. But does this impulse to seek a member of the opposite sex, which Moll has called the impulse of contrectation, satisfy a genuine need other than the need for ejaculation which can be satisfied more easily in other ways? We have seen that it is the threat of loneliness and of hunger which this seemed to imply which is largely responsible for the child's longing for its mother.[1] In the adult this impulse is possibly an irrelevant avoidance of a threat which has lost its meaning. This and similar irrelevant avoidances may have been selected to build up the contrectative impulses of the race. If they are irrelevant their abolition would require a degree of self-knowledge which is at present unthinkable. But the possibility of such an antagonism between instinct and intelligence remains.

The second example concerns the instincts of self-which we have so far alone considered. It might, however, involve new dangers of its own of an opposite type. For there is no more guarantee that the train of reactions which involves most pleasure must be in the interests of the race than there is that the train which involves least pain has this attribute.

[1] *Cf.* Chap. ii, 121 ; Chap. iii, 221 ; chap. v, 22.

preservation. Removal reactions are determined by needs. They continue until the need ceases, so that their aim may be said to be the removal of needs. From the point of view of evolution, the best removal is that which most promotes the survival of the species. But from the individual's point of view it would seem to be the reaction that most quickly removes the need which is the best. Now the quickest and most final method by which an individual can remove his needs is to put his head in a gas-oven or to adopt some other equally painless method of self-extermination. He does not do so, partly because he thinks in terms of seekings rather than of removals, and partly, because of the instinct of self-preservation.[1] The impulse of self-preservation is ultimately the impulse to avoid the pain of injuries. Although death is painless it is to most of us a false threat of pain. But even those who are convinced that there is no pain in death do not often kill themselves. However great their need they remain obsessed by the image of the means which evolution has determined that they shall seek in order to remove it, and do not take the short cut which their intelligence suggests.

The danger that knowledge will destroy instincts is of course remote. But it is just possible that the individualists of the future not only may be too lazy to propagate their species, but that they may even discover that the lethal chamber is an easier and more permanent means to the removal of their needs than the circuitous method of sowing, reaping, harvesting,

[1] *Cf.* Chap. iii, 17, 226; iv, 21.

eating, and copulating, which they now employ. If this should ever come to pass, the universe will be clear for the growth of some species of ant or termite whose instincts are less sullied by intelligence.

If man could become truly negatively hedonistic and capable of seeking only the shortest route to the removal of his needs and injuries, his unpleasures and his pains, it seems to me inevitable that he would ultimately learn to seek only his painless extinction. But he is not solely negatively hedonistic, or rather he is unlikely ever to discover the shortest route to his complete and utter satiation. Certain false threats and irrelevant fears will remain with him as an entailed estate, which he may recognize intellectually but not emotionally, and which will prevent him from escaping from his needs except by the circuitous routes which serve not his purpose but the continuation of the race. For this reason I do not think that instincts have anything to fear from the growth of self-knowledge.

If the instinct of self-preservation remains strong in the individual it is natural that he will reconcile his inevitable extinction by transferring this desire to the race. It will become for him a matter of grave concern to provide a new refuge for his species in another planet, when the earth has become cold and uninhabitable, or in another solar system when the sun itself has shared a similar fate, and even to foresee some hope of immortality in spite of the second law of thermodynamics which seems to doom the entire universe to destruction.

The first two cataclysms could probably be avoided

with sufficient mechanical ingenuity, so that the racial altruist who has projected his fear of death upon his species would wish for a social system that promoted a knowledge of pure physics and its applications, and would deplore all tendencies to play after our past labours in communistic garden cities, and so to waste the few billion years of grace which precedes the destruction of the earth.[1]

Such a method of escaping from the doom of the earth involves a modification of our environment; it is an alloplastic adaptation. But if we are to escape a final and still remoter destruction, our adaptations must be autoplastic also, they must involve a modification of ourselves. So far, we have developed from the amoeba by means of variations which we have not influenced and selections which we have not controlled. But the time is coming when we may be able surgically to influence the chromosomes and promote any type we choose, and already we could purposefully select spontaneous variations if we were agreed upon what variations to select, and upon the method of selecting them. Therefore, it is becoming important to decide the direction in which we wish to influence evolution.

It is, of course, impossible for us to imagine that it would be pleasant to be organisms entirely unlike ourselves. Our amoeboid ancestors would probably have agreed that their simple aquatic life was preferable to our more troubled existence. Similarly it is

[1] Haldane, in an interesting story of the end of the world, imagines the Sidereal colonists, who escaped from the earth, to have been dominated by this kind of racial altruism.

difficult to imagine ourselves with pleasure as the bodiless cerebra which we may some day become. The preferences of the amoeba were of no importance, for they did not control evolution. With us, however, the case is different, for we can control our future. If we prefer to remain unchanged or to degenerate into less intelligent and more appetitive types we can do so. But if we wish to live for ever, we must continue to adapt ourselves to our environment as well as our environment to ourselves, and we must further foresee and anticipate the adaptations which one day will be necessary.

If we self-consciously follow out some such racial ambition as I have suggested, it seems possible that the destiny of man will be a solitary exception to the general degradation of inanimate matter. While the rest of the universe is breaking up into simpler and ever simpler particles, man may conceivably continue that process of increasing complication which the organic world, as an infinitesimal exception to the inorganic, has already pursued for so long, and he may end as a single gigantic brain which operates throughout the ages without the least dissipation of its remaining energy. Since the rest of the universe would have disappeared, this brain would have no necessity for organs of locomotion or perception ; since it would conserve its own energy, it would take no nourishment ; and since it would be immortal, it would not need to reproduce itself. Its correlated mental activities would be unthinkable to us. But though it would have no external perceptions and no desires which it could not fulfil autonomously, it could still narcissistically enjoy an acute awareness of itself. It would be like the Spinozistic God, pure Being, engaged eternally in the contemplation of its own perfection. But the human philosopher may legitimately wonder whether this or race extinction is the more preferable goal.

4. *The value of psychology.*

In the last three sections we have considered some of the effects which might be expected of psychology. In this we shall discuss its value.

I suppose that the fundamental definition of value is that value is the property of anything which facilitates the satisfaction of desires. In other words, anything is valuable which assists the removal or avoidance of injuries and needs.

Thus, means or anything which facilitates the seeking of means, has value. Knowledge of physics is valuable because it is often a condition to the attainment of means. It gives us motor cars, ships, and aeroplanes to carry us quickly to the things and people we desire to see, electric light and labour-saving houses to reduce our drudgery, and so puts us in ever closer contact with the things we think we want.

A part of the value of psychology is of a similar nature, for it does to persons what physics does to things. It teaches us to act on them so that they will react in what we believe to be our interests. Thus the successful statesman, industrialist, and seducer must all possess some knowledge of psychology.

A greater value of psychology lies, not in that it facilitates the attainment of the means we already consciously desire, but in that it frees inhibited impulses. Irrelevant inhibitions, that is, irrelevant avoidances opposed to adequate seekings, are responsible for the chief deprivations of this life. Only when these are destroyed by self-knowledge can needs be removed which were previously unsatisfied.

The positive function of psychology of freeing inhibited desires is, however, secondary to the negative function of destroying inhibitions, and this is but a special case of its still more general function of destroying all irrelevant and inadequate impulses. It may, like other sciences, help to satisfy conscious impulses ; it may free those which are not conscious, and thereby permit their satisfaction, and because it can do these things it has value. But it is not only valuable because it satisfies impulses, but also because it destroys them.

No one would deny that anything which destroys a fear has value. But what of a science which destroys a cherished positive desire ? A neurotic does not object to the loss of his anxiety. But the pervert, in analysis, will struggle tenaciously against the loss of his perversion. We have seen that it is very difficult to decide what are adequate and what inadequate desires. It is possible that many of the things which we most value do not remove real needs, and would be devaluated by an analysis which was sufficiently exhaustive. Those who fear such consequences misunderstand the possible result. They cannot imagine that they could cease to like something which they now desire, and they think that they are threatened with the loss of some object or activity while the desire for it remains. Like the child, they cannot imagine that they could ever cease to love their toys. But even if psychology should teach us to approximate to the Buddhist ideal, it would still have value. For value is a property of anything which facilitates the satisfaction of desires. And desires are also satisfied when they are destroyed.

INDEX

P

Printed and bound by CPI Group (UK) Ltd, Croydon, CR0 4YY

01/11/2024

01782632-0008